OCULAR PATHOLOGY

A COLOR ATLAS

MYRON YANOFF MD, FACA
Professor of Ophthalmology and Pathology
University of Pennsylvania School of Medicine and Scheie Eye Institute
Former Director and Chairman, Department of Ophthalmology
University of Pennsylvania and Scheie Eye Institute

BEN S. FINE MD
Research Associate, Department of Ophthalmic Pathology
Armed Forces Institute of Pathology
Associate Research Professor of Ophthalmology
The George Washington University
Senior Attending Ophthalmologist
The Washington Hospital Center
Washington DC
Clinical Professor of Pathology
Uniformed Services
University of the Health Sciences
Bethesda, MD

J.B. LIPPINCOTT COMPANY • PHILADELPHIA
GOWER MEDICAL PUBLISHING • NEW YORK • LONDON

Distributed in the USA and Canada by:
J.B. Lippincott Company
East Washington Square
Philadelphia, PA 19105, USA

Distributed in all countries except the USA and Canada by:
Harper & Row Publishers Inc. International Division
10 East 53rd Street
New York, NY 10022, USA

Library of Congress Cataloging-in-Publication Data

Yanoff, Myron.
    Ocular pathology.
    Companion v. to: Ocular pathology : a text and atlas /
Myron Yanoff, Ben S. Fine. 2nd ed. © 1982.
    Includes bibliographies and index.
    1. Eye–Diseases and defects—Atlases. 2. Eye—
Wounds and injuries–Atlases. I. Fine, Ben S.,
1928–   . II. Title. [DNLM: 1. Eye Diseases—
pathology—atlases. WW 17 Y24o]
RE50.Y36 1982   Suppl   617.7′1   87-11965
ISBN 0 397 44659-4

British Library Cataloging in Publication Data

Yanoff, Myron
    Ocular Pathology: a color atlas
    1. Eye-Diseases and defects
    I. Title   II. Fine, Ben S.
    617.7′1   RE46
    ISBN 0-397-44659-4

Project Editor   Valerie Neal
Illustrators   Alan Landau and Carol Kalafatic
Art Director   Jill Feltham
Design   Jessica Stockholder

Printed in Singapore by Imago Productions (FE) PTE Ltd

We dedicate this book to the memory of Paul Henkind MD, PhD, who accomplished a prodigious amount himself, and who stimulated so many to do more than they would have otherwise. Paul's own words best convey his uniqueness:

I do not wish to be in a different time or a different place
Nor wish a different mind or a different face
The challenge within is simply to be the man in me.

PREFACE

Tissues should be viewed in color. There is something quite special about looking through a microscope at otherwise invisible structures, now splashed in color and vividly outlined. Why then are pictures in textbooks almost always in black and white? Until recently, both price and difficulty in high-quality color reproduction have been the limiting factors. Fortunately, our publishers have offered us excellent color reproduction at an affordable price. We, therefore, set about to prepare a highly selective color atlas of ocular pathology that would serve as companion to our textbook, *Ocular Pathology: A Text and Atlas*. The material presented has been chosen because it is common, it is important, or it is new. The selection of material for the bibliography at the end of each chapter was arbitrary; these references should serve only as an introductory guide.

The format here is similar to that used in *Ocular Pathology: A Text and Atlas*. This book is divided into 18 chapters covering basic principles, congenital and systemic diseases, inflammations and tumors, generalized ocular disorders, and more specific abnormalities of the various ocular tissues. Each chapter has a brief introduction that provides an overview of the subject matter. The introduction is then followed by a series of illustrations. Tabular figures introduce each subject area, listing important entities. These are followed by a series of photographic figures that illustrate selected entities. The entities are presented, wherever possible, in a clinicopathologic fashion.

Because the total number of illustrations had to be limited in order to contain the size and cost of the book, and because we wanted to utilize as many color illustrations as possible, black and white reproductions used in *Ocular Pathology: A Text and Atlas* are included here only on rare occasions. These include electron micrographs, fluorescein angiograms, plus CT and magnetic resonance images.

Finally, a few words on why we have produced another book on eye pathology. The 1980s have seen the publication of more textbooks on eye pathology than the preceding 3 decades. These textbooks have grown considerably in size and complexity. Certainly, another encyclopedic book is not now needed. What is required is brevity and color illustrations. Our hope is that *Ocular Pathology: A Color Atlas* will give the student (from resident to practicing ophthalmologist and pathologist) a comprehensive overview and understanding of ocular pathology in a concise, interesting format. For a more in-depth review, the reader is referred to *Ocular Pathology: A Text and Atlas* and any other of the numerous pathology textbooks published over the last few years.

As always, we are greatly indebted to our mentor, Lorenz E. Zimmerman MD, who continues to be an inspiration to us as a teacher and leader in ophthalmic pathology. Without his influence this and our previous books would not have been written. We also would like to acknowledge David Barsky MD, for his pioneering work in producing a color atlas of eye pathology in 1966. J. Valerie Neal, PhD, our editor at Gower Medical Publishing, did a superb job both in editing the entire manuscript and in prodding us gently to keep us on schedule. Alan Landau and Carol Kalafatic translated our very rough sketches and line drawings into works of art. Jessica Stockholder designed all of the pages and made certain that everything fit together and worked visually. Most of all, we thank Karin L. Yanoff, Fruma I. Fine, and our children for their loving help and tolerance during our preparation of this book.

Myron Yanoff MD
Ben S. Fine MD

CONTENTS

BASIC PRINCIPLES OF PATHOLOGY 1

A tissue responds to a noxious stimulus by a process called inflammation. Generally, inflammation may be considered as a nonspecific or specific immune reaction to a foreign agent. The noxious stimulus or foreign agent may be infectious or noninfectious, and any individual tissue or some combination of tissues may be affected.

Both noninfectious agents, such as chemicals or allergens, or infectious agents, such as bacteria and fungi, may induce inflammation. Inflammation may be endogenous or exogenous. Endogenous inflammation is caused by a process occurring in the eye itself, such as phacolytic glaucoma in which leaking denatured lens protein induces a macrophagic inflammatory reaction. Exogenous inflammation is caused by a process occurring at a remote site, an example of which is bacterial endocarditis sending emboli to the retina, resulting in infectious retinitis.

The inflammatory process consists of both cellular components and chemical mediators. The interaction of different factors, including histamine, serotonin, kinins, and others, results in the cardinal signs of inflammation—redness, heat, edema, pain,

and loss of function. An inflammatory reaction may be divided into an acute phase, a subacute or intermediate phase, and a chronic phase. The subacute or intermediate phase is most closely related to the immune reaction.

The chronic phase may be divided into nongranulomatous and granulomatous types. The nongranulomatous type is characterized by the presence of lymphocytes and plasma cells. A cause for this type of inflammation usually is not found. The granulomatous type is characterized by the presence of epithelioid cells, and the cause (e.g., tuberculosis and toxoplasmosis) often is found. The granulomatous type often shows inflammatory giant cells, such as foreign body, Langhans, and Touton giant cells. The inflammatory pattern may be helpful in identifying a cause. For example, a diffuse granulomatous pattern is seen in sympathetic uveitis, a discrete pattern in sarcoidosis, and a zonal pattern in phacoanaphylactic endophthalmitis.

The entities that cause inflammation will be illustrated in the appropriate chapters. Here concepts of humoral and cellular immunity are illustrated.

FIG. 1.1 TYPES OF INFLAMMATION

Acute (exudative)	Subacute (intermediate)	Chronic (proliferative)
Polymorphonuclear leukocytes	Healing	Nongranulomatous: lymphocytes and plasma cells
Mast cells and eosinophils	Chronicity	Granulomatous: epithelioid cells

FIG. 1.2 CELLS INVOLVED IN ACUTE INFLAMMATION

Polymorphonuclear leukocyte

Bone-marrow-derived

First line of cellular defense

Drawn to site by chemotaxis

Marginate in venules by adhering to wall junction

Emigrate between endothelial cells into tissue

Remove noxious agents (bacteria) by phagocytosis and lysosomal digestion

Eosinophilic leukocyte

Bone-marrow-derived

Found in allergic and parasitic conditions

Phagocytic

Granules contain proteolytic enzymes

Mast cell (basophilic leukocyte)

Fixed tissue cells

Elaborate heparin and histamine

Basophils can be considered circulating mast cells

FIG. 1.3 GRANULATION TISSUE INVOLVED IN SUBACUTE INFLAMMATION

Acute and chronic inflammatory cells
Fibroblasts

Vascular endothelial cells

FIG. 1.4 TYPES OF CHRONIC INFLAMMATION

Granulomatous

Epithelioid cells necessary for diagnosis

Giant cells often present

Good chance of finding cause

Nongranulomatous

Lymphocyte (competent immunocyte)

B lymphocyte

T lymphocyte

Plasma cell

Rarely find a cause

FIG. 1.5 COMPETENT IMMUNOCYTES SEEN IN CHRONIC INFLAMMATION

B Lymphocyte

Bone-marrow derived

Active in humoral immunity

Source of immunoglobulin

Plasma cell precursor

Function: immunity to bacteria and neutralization of toxins

T Lymphocyte

Modified by thymus gland

Active in cell-mediated immunity

Produce a variety of lymphokines

Function: immunity to mycobacteria, viruses, fungi; and graft rejection

FIG 1.6 MACROPHAGE (HISTIOCYTE) SEEN IN
CHRONIC INFLAMMATION

Circulating monocytes and tissue histiocytes

Chief phagocyte

Processes antigen for lymphocytes in immune reaction

Epithelioid cell and giant cell precursor

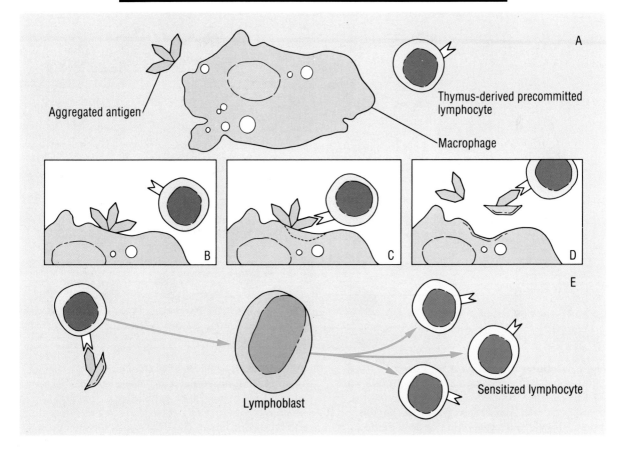

Fig. 1.7 Cellular Immunity. A The participants in the cellular immune response include the thymus-derived precommitted lymphocyte (T-cell), bone-marrow-derived monocyte (macrophage), and the aggregated antigens. **B** Aggregated antigen is seen attaching to the surface of the macrophage. **C** The T-cell is shown as it attaches to the aggregated antigen. **D** The substance originating in the macrophage passes into the T-cell, which is attached to the antigen. **E** The combined T-cell, antigen, and macrophagic material causes the T-cell to enlarge into a lymphoblast. Sensitized, or committed, T-lymphocytes arise from lymphoblasts.

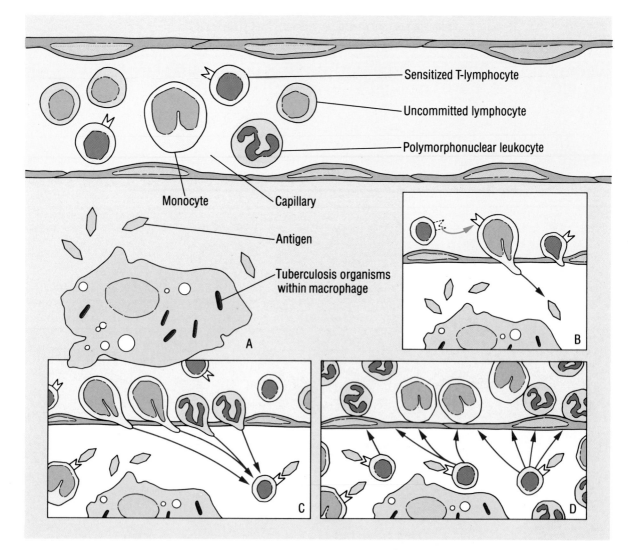

Fig. 1.8 Cellular Immunity. A Sensitized T-lymphocytes (SL) are seen in a capillary. Along with the SL are other leukocytes, including monocytes, at an antigenic site. A macrophage, which contains tubercle bacilli, and antigen may be seen in the surrounding tissue. **B** Monocytes become sensitized when cytophilic antibody from SL is transferred to them. They migrate toward the antigenic stimulus. **C** Biologically active molecules, which cause the monocytes and leukocytes to travel to the area, are released by SL when they have encountered a specific antigen. **D** Monocytes arriving at the site are immobilized by migration-inhibitory factor (MIF), which is released by SL, which also releases cytotoxin and mitogenic factor. Cytotoxin causes tissue necrosis (caseation), and mitogenic factor causes proliferation of cells. Some of these cells undergo transformation, becoming epithelioid cells causing the formation of a tuberculoma.

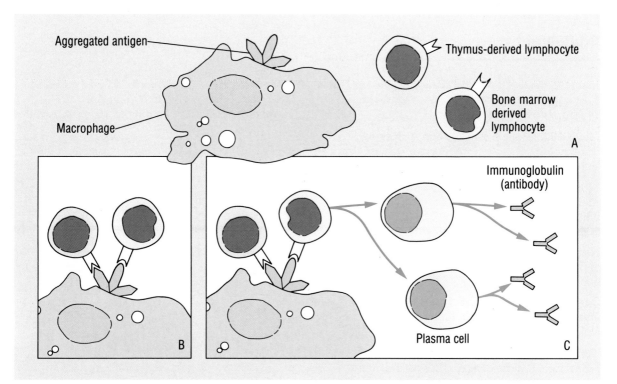

Fig. 1.9 Humoral Immunity. A, B Four prerequisites for immunoglobulin formation are demonstrated including thymus-derived lymphocyte (T-cell), thymus-independent bone-marrow-derived lymphocyte (B-cell), bone-marrow-derived monocyte (macrophage), and aggregated antigen. In **A**, aggregated antigens are seen attached to macrophages. In **B**, T- and B-cells are seen attached to different determinants on the aggregated antigen. **C** Cooperative interaction that occurs between the T- and B-cells causes the B-cells to differentiate into plasma cells.

FIG. 1.10 NONINFLAMMATORY CELLULAR AND TISSUE REACTIONS

Hypertrophy—increased size of individual cells

Hyperplasia—increased number of individual cells

Aplasia—lack of embryologic development of a tissue

Hypoplasia—arrest of embryologic development of a tissue

Metaplasia—transformation of one type of tissue into another

Atrophy—decrease in size of fully developed tissue

Neoplasia—continuous, unregulated increase in cells in a tissue

Degeneration—change in a tissue resulting from previous diseases

Dystrophy—primary inheritable disorder

Necrosis—death of cells

Calcification

Bibliography

Jakobiec FA, Lefkowitch J, Knowles DM: B- and T-lymphocytes in ocular disease. Ophthalmology 91:635, 1984.

James DG, Graham E, Hamblin A: Review. Immunology of multisystem ocular disease. Surv Ophthalmol 30:155, 1985.

Milanese C, Richardson NE, Reinherz EL: Identification of a T helper cell-derived lymphokine that activates resting T lymphocytes. Science 231:1118, 1986.

Nago K, Yukoro K, Aaronson SA: Continuous lines of basophil/mast cells derived from normal mouse bone marrow. Science 212:333, 1981.

Quigley HA, Kenyon KR: Russell bodies and plasma cells in human conjunctiva. Am J Ophthalmol 76:957, 1973.

Turk JL: Immunologic and nonimmunologic activation of macrophages. J Invest Dermatol 74:301, 1980.

Turner RR, Egbert P, Warnke RA: Lymphocytic infiltrates of the conjunctiva and orbit: immunohistochemical staining of 16 cases. Am J Clin Pathol 81:447, 1984.

Weiss SJ, et al: Oxidative autoactivation of latent collagenase by human neutrophils. Science 227:747, 1985.

Williams GT, Williams WJ: Granulomatous inflammation—a review. J Clin Pathol 36:723, 1983.

Zimmerman LE: Ocular lesions of juvenile xanthogranuloma. Nevoxanthoendothelioma. Trans Am Acad Ophthalmol Otolaryngol 69:412, 1965.

CONGENITAL ANOMALIES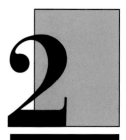

Congenital ocular anomalies that are associated with systemic anomalies may have a variety of causes. Broadly, the causes may be subdivided into:
- chromosomal aberrations;
- infectious embryopathies;
- drug embryopathies;
- phakomatoses;
- and other entities.

In chromosomal aberrations, the normal total number of chromosomes (44 autosomes and 2 sex chromosomes) may be present, but individual chromosomes may have structural alterations, as occurs in the chromosome 18 deletion defect, in which there is a deletion of one of the arms of the chromosome. Alternatively, the total number of chromosomes may be abnormal, too few (45) as is seen in Turner syndrome, or too many (47) as in Down's syndrome. Other aberrations, such as mosaicism, also occur.

Infectious embryopathies, such as rubella and toxoplasmosis, result from infection of the embryo *in utero*, which is especially susceptible during the first trimester of gestation. Similarly, drug embryopathies are caused by substances, such as thalidomide, that cross the blood–placental barrier from mother to fetus, adversely affecting the embryo. Again, the fetus is most susceptible during the first trimester of gestation.

The phakomatoses are a group of congenital tumors of genetic origin, which have in common the characteristic of disseminated hamartomas, usually benign. In an individual phakomatosis, the hamartomas tend to affect one type of tissue predominantly; blood vessels in meningocutaneous angiomatoses (Sturge–Weber syndrome), and peripheral nerves in neurofibromatosis.

Many other congenital ocular and systemic anomalies, similar to the phakomatoses, have a genetic origin but are not easily classified in groups. Still other anomalies seem to occur by chance, and have no known cause.

FIG. 2.1 CHROMOSOMAL ABERRATIONS SEEN IN CONGENITAL ANOMALIES

Defect in number	Deletion defect (46 chromosomes)	Mosaicism
Trisomy (47 chromosomes)	Chromosome 5 (*cri-du-chat* syndrome)	Two or more populations of karyotypically distinct chromosomes
Trisomy 13	Chromosome 13 (may be associated with retinoblastoma)	
Trisomy 18	Chromosome 18	
Trisomy 21 (Downs's syndrome)		
Triploidy (69 chromosomes)		
Turner syndrome (45 chromosomes)		

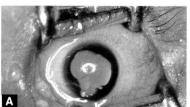

Fig. 2.2   Trisomy 13. A An inferior nasal iris coloboma and leukokoria are present. **B** A coloboma of the ciliary body is filled with mesenchymal tissue containing cartilage. Note the retinal dysplasia. Generally, in trisomy 13 cartilage is present in microphthalmic eyes smaller than 10 mm in size. (**A**, courtesy of Dr. DB Schaffer; **B**, case reported in Hoepner J, Yanoff M, 1972.)

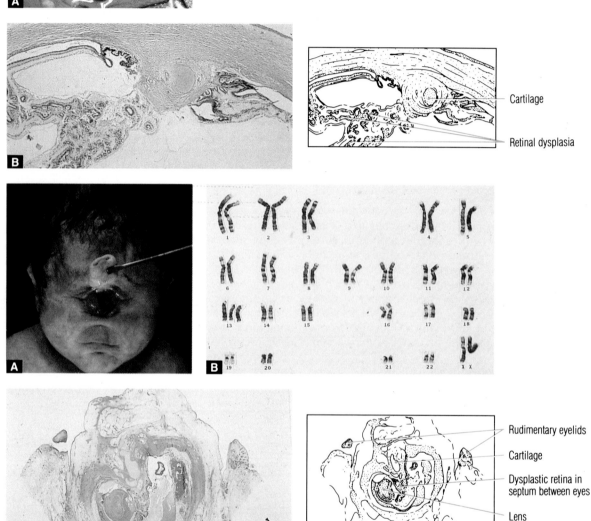

Cartilage

Retinal dysplasia

Rudimentary eyelids

Cartilage

Dysplastic retina in septum between eyes

Lens

Fig. 2.3   Trisomy 13. A The patient was born with clinical cyclops. When the proboscis is lifted, a single pseudo-orbit is seen clinically. Note the fairly well formed eyelids under the proboscis. **B** Karyotype from the same patient shows an extra chromosome (three instead of two) in the 13 group. **C** Histologic section shows that the condition is not true cyclops (a single eye), but the more commonly seen synophthalmos (partial fusion of the two eyes).

FIG. 2.4 MORBID EMBRYOPATHIES SEEN IN CONGENITAL ANOMALIES

Infectious embryopathies
Toxoplasmosis
Cytomegalic inclusion disease
Congenital rubella syndrome
Congenital syphilis

Drug embryopathies
Thalidomide
Lysergic acid diethylamide (LSD)

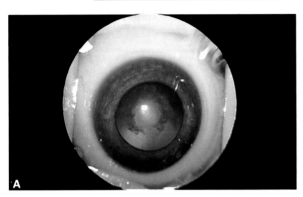

Fig. 2.5 Rubella. A A dense nuclear cataract is seen in the pupillary red reflex, surrounded by a less dense cortical cataract. Congenital infection with rubella is characterized by ocular and cardiovascular abnormalities and deafness. The most common ocular finding is a "salt and pepper" fundus, followed by cataract. **B** Histologic section shows a cataractous lens. **C** High magnification shows retention of the nuclei within the fetal nucleus of the lens. (**A**, courtesy of Dr. DB Schaffer.)

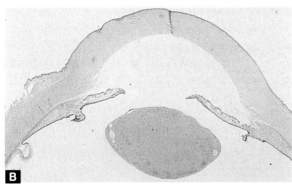

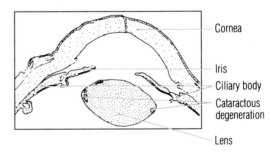

Cornea
Iris
Ciliary body
Cataractous degeneration
Lens

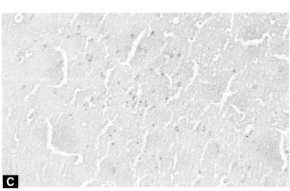

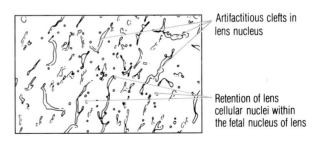

Artifactitious clefts in lens nucleus

Retention of lens cellular nuclei within the fetal nucleus of lens

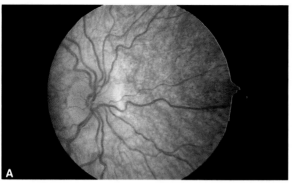

Fig. 2.6   Rubella. A Both fine and coarse pigmentation are present in the fundus at the level of the retinal pigment epithelium (RPE). **B** Histologic section shows that the RPE is hypertrophied in this region whereas in other regions, shown in **C**, the pigment epithelium is atrophic and has lost most of its pigment. It is the alternating areas of hypertrophy and atrophy of the RPE that give rise to the clinical picture of "salt and pepper" fundus. (**A**, courtesy of Dr. DB Schaffer.)

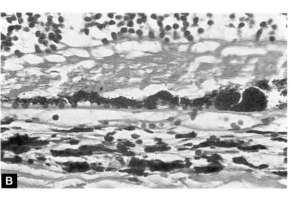

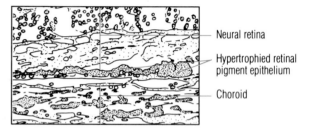

Neural retina

Hypertrophied retinal pigment epithelium

Choroid

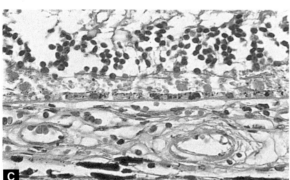

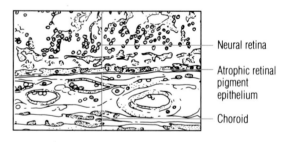

Neural retina

Atrophic retinal pigment epithelium

Choroid

FIG. 2.7 PHAKOMATOSES

Angiomatosis retinae (von Hippel's disease)
Meningocutaneous angiomatosis (Sturge–Weber syndrome)
Neurofibromatosis (von Recklinghausen's disease)
Tuberous sclerosis (Bourneville's disease)
Ataxia telangiectasia (Louis–Bar syndrome)
Arteriovenous communication of retina and brain
   (Wyburn–Mason syndrome)

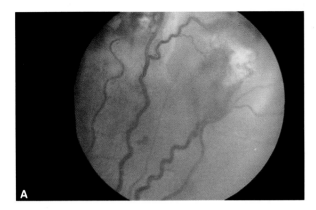

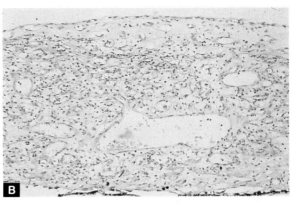

Fig. 2.8 von Hippel's Disease. A Superiorly, two round retinal lesions associated with von Hippel's disease (angiomatosis retinae) are apparent along with feeder vessels. B Histologic section shows two distinct types of cells: endothelial cells lining the numerous capillaries; and, present between the capillaries, stromal cells which are derived from vascular endothelium that appear "foamy". (B, courtesy of Dr. DH Nicholson.)

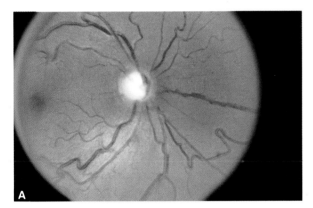

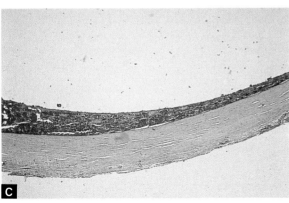

Fig. 2.9 Sturge–Weber Syndrome. A The fundus shows the characteristic bright red appearance of the involved eye, caused by the choroidal hemangioma, as well as the enlarged optic nerve cup, secondary to increased intraocular pressure in that eye. B The normal fundus of the patient's left eye is shown for comparison. C In another case, the choroid is diffusely involved by a cavernous hemangioma. When a choroidal hemangioma occurs in the Sturge–Weber patient, it is diffuse, large, and difficult to distinguish from any normal choroid that might be present. When it occurs in a patient without the syndrome, it is focal, small, and easy to distinguish from the surrounding normal choroid. (C, courtesy of Dr. R Cordero-Moreno, from *Ocular Pathology*, 2nd edn, by M Yanoff and BS Fine.)

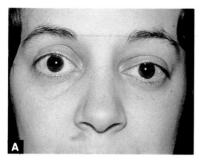
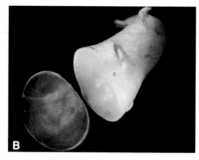
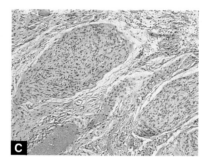

Fig. 2.10   Neurofibromatosis A. A neurofibroma is enlarging the left upper lid. The neurofibroma was removed. **B** The gross specimen shows a markedly enlarged nerve. A thin slice of the nerve is present at the bottom left. **C** Histologic section from another case shows the markedly enlarged nerves in neurofibromatosis of the orbit. (**A**, courtesy of Dr. WC Frayer.)

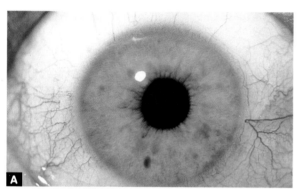

Fig. 2.11   Neurofibromatosis. A Iris shows multiple small spider-like melanocytic nevi, characteristic of neurofibromatosis. **B** The iris nevi are caused by collections of nevus cells. **C** The choroid is markedly thickened by the hamartomatous process. Note thickened nerves in sclera. Numerous structures such as neural rosettes, tactile nerve endings and nevi may be found.

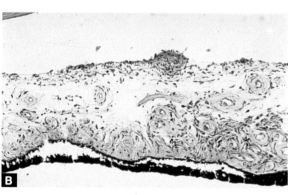
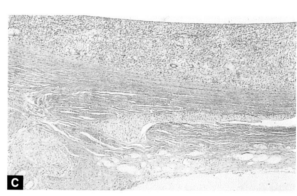

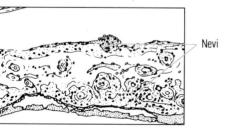

Nevi

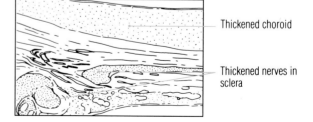

Thickened choroid

Thickened nerves in sclera

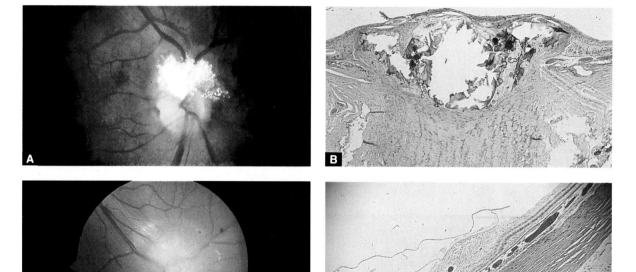

Fig. 2.12   Tuberous Sclerosis. A Fundus shows typical mulberry lesion involving the superior part of the optic nerve. **B** Histologic section of another case shows a giant drusen of the optic nerve. **C** The lesion, as seen in the fundus of a young child before it grows into the mulberry configuration, is quite smooth and resembles a retinoblastoma. **D** Histologic section of an early lesion shows no calcification but simply a proliferation of glial tissue. (**A**, from *Ocular Pathology*, 2nd edn, by M Yanoff and BS Fine. **C**, courtesy of Dr. DB Schaffer.)

FIG. 2.13 ASSORTED CONDITIONS SEEN IN CONGENITAL ANOMALIES

Anencephaly (absence of cranial vault)

Anophthalmos (absence of eye)

Microphthalmos (eye less than 15 mm in greatest diameter at birth)

Lowe's syndrome (oculocerebrorenal syndrome, systemic acidosis, organic aciduria, renal rickets, congenital cataract, glaucoma)

Miller's syndrome (oculocerebrorenal syndrome, Wilm's tumor, aniridia, genitourinary anomalies)

Leigh's syndrome (subacute necrotizing encephalomyelopathy)

de Lange syndrome (mental and growth retardation, characteristic facial appearance, multiple skeletal abnormalities, low-pitched cry)

Meckel syndrome (posterior encephalocele, polydactyly, polycystic kidney)

Menkes' disease (defect in copper absorption, cerebral degeneration, arterial changes, sparse brittle scalp hair)

Dwarfism (many types)

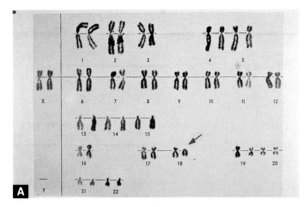

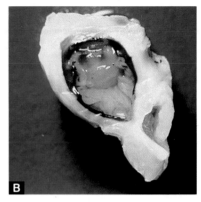

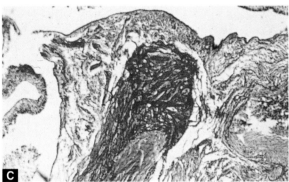

Fig. 2.14 Microphthalmos. A Parts of the long and short arms of one of the chromosomes in the 18 group are missing (arrow) in this karyotype. The entity is called chromosome 18 deletion defect. The patient had bilateral microphthalmos with cyst. **B** The opened gross specimen of the patient's left eye shows a small eye and a contiguous cyst (the right eye was quite similar). **C** Smooth muscle found in the choroid near the optic nerve is bright red when treated with the trichrome stain. (Case reported in Yanoff M et al, 1970.)

Bibliography

Brownstein S, Little JM: Ocular neurofibromatosis. Ophthalmology 90:1595, 1983.

Cibis GW, Tripathi RC, Tripathi BJ: Glaucoma in Sturge–Weber syndrome. Ophthalmology 91:1061, 1984.

Hardwig P, Robertson DM: von Hippel–Lindau disease: a familial, often lethal, multi-system phakomatosis. Ophthalmology 91:263, 1984.

Hoepner J, Yanoff M: Ocular anomalies in trisomy 13-15: an analysis of 13 eyes with two new findings. Am J Ophthalmol 74:729, 1972.

Krohel GB, et al: Localized orbital neurofibromas. Am J Ophthalmol 100:458, 1985.

Mets MB, Maumenee IH: Review. The eye and the chromosome. Surv Ophthalmol 28:20, 1983.

Williams R, Taylor D: Review. Tuberous sclerosis. Surv Ophthalmol 30:143, 1985.

Yanoff M, Rorke LB, Niederer BS: Ocular and cerebral abnormalities in chromosome 18 deletion defect. Am J Ophthalmol 70:391, 1970.

Yanoff M, Schaffer DB, Scheie HG: Rubella ocular syndrome—clinical significance of viral and pathologic studies. Trans Am Acad Ophthalmol Otolaryngol 72:896, 1968.

NONGRANULOMATOUS INFLAMMATION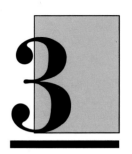

Nongranulomatous inflammation may be designated either suppurative or nonsuppurative. The suppurative form, which has an acute onset and is characterized by the formation of pus, may be manifested in ocular congestion, chemosis, hazy media, hypopyon, pain, and exophthalmos. The polymorphonuclear leukocyte is the predominant inflammatory cell. A reaction in nongranulomatous inflammation may be exogenous, secondary to the presence of an intraocular foreign body following a penetrating or perforating injury to the eye; or endogenous, an example of which is necrosis of a uveal melanoma leading to marked endophthalmitis. Nongranulomatous inflammation also may be manifested in the following ways:

- endophthalmitis—the inflammation of one or more coats of the eye and adjacent cavities;
- panophthalmitis—inflammation of one or more coats of the eye and adjacent cavities plus scleral involvement and spread to orbital tissue.

Nonsuppurative nongranulomatous inflammation may be acute or chronic. The acute type is characterized by inflammation in which the polymorphonuclear leukocyte is the predominant cell, as seen in cellulitis secondary to *Streptococcus hemolyticus* infection. The acute type does not lead to suppuration or pus formation. Lymphocytes and plasma cells also may be the predominant cell types, as seen in acute iritis.

In the chronic type of nongranulomatous inflammation, the plasma cell and the lymphocyte usually predominate, as seen in the "garden variety" type of uveitis. Many different entities can cause a nongranulomatous inflammation, including traumatic iridocyclitis, heterochromic iridocyclitis (Fuchs), rheumatoid arthritis, and various idiopathic diseases. Less common causes include Behçet's syndrome, Reiter's syndrome, pars planitis, and others. Although the list of possible causes is long, in general, in any given patient, a cause is rarely found for chronic nonsuppurative nongranulomatous inflammation.

The aftermaths or sequelae of nongranulomatous inflammation are numerous and span the spectrum from minor problems to major disorders.

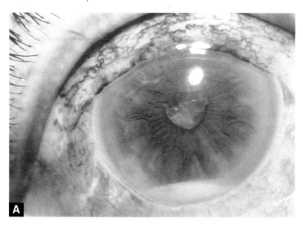

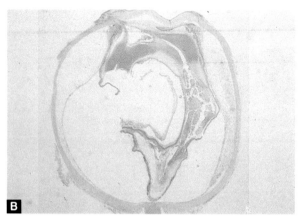

Fig. 3.1 Endophthalmitis. A The patient developed "sterile" endophthalmitis after undergoing extracapsular cataract extraction and a posterior chamber lens implant. Note the hypopyon. **B** Another patient developed bacterial endophthalmitis following intracapsular cataract extraction. The diffuse abscess seen filling the vitreous cavity is characteristic of bacterial infection (fungal infection usually causes multiple tiny abscesses). The retina and its adjacent cavity, the vitreous, are involved but the choroid and sclera are spared.

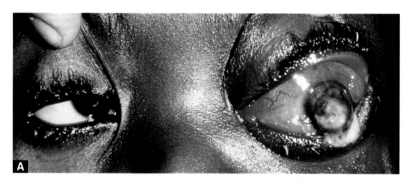

Fig. 3.2 Panophthalmitis. A The patient had a regular measles infection and subsequently developed pain and inflammation in the left eye that led to panophthalmitis and corneal perforation. **B** Histologic section shows the corneal perforation. The vitreous body, adjacent retina, choroid, and sclera are all involved, and the inflammation extends through the coats of the eye into the episcleral tissue. (**A**, courtesy of Dr. RE Shannon.)

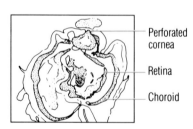

Perforated cornea

Retina

Choroid

Exogenous
Iridocyclitis secondary to keratitis or corneal ulcer
Nonsurgical or surgical trauma
Endogenous
Metastatic septic emboli
Necrosis of uveal melanoma
Spread from sinus inflammation
Behçet's syndrome

Oral ulceration—aphthous stomatitis

Genital ulceration

Ocular inflammation—recurrent iridocyclitis, hypopyon, and retinal necrosis

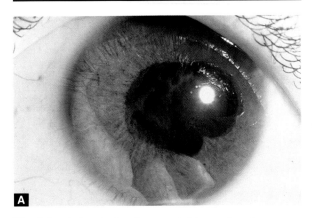

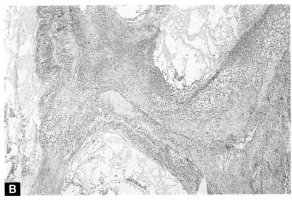

Fig. 3.5   Behçet's Syndrome. A The patient has a hypopyon. Note the posterior synechiae, a sign of the recurrent iridocyclitis in this patient. **B** A histologic section shows necrosis and perivasculitis of the retina. An organizing cyclitic membrane has caused a detachment of the retina. (**A**, from *Ocular Pathology*, 2nd edn, by M Yanoff and BS Fine; (**B**, case presented by Dr. TA Makley at the Verhoeff Society in 1976.)

FIG. 3.6 CAUSES OF NONSUPPURATIVE INFLAMMATION

Exogenous
Blunt trauma
Perforating trauma
Endogenous
Idiopathic ("garden variety" uveitis) most common
Associated with systemic diseases
Rheumatoid arthritis
Reiter syndrome (nonbacterial urethritis, conjunctivitis or iridocyclitis, and arthritis)
Crohn's disease
Whipple's disease

Viral
Rubella
Herpes simplex and *zoster*
Subacute sclerosing panencephalitis (chronic, progressive CNS disease in childhood caused by the measles virus, usually 5 to 7 years after the primary measles infection)

Nonsystemic syndromes
Uveal effusion
Pars planitis
Glaucomatocyclitic crisis (Posner–Schlossman syndrome)
Heterochromic iridocyclitis (Fuchs)

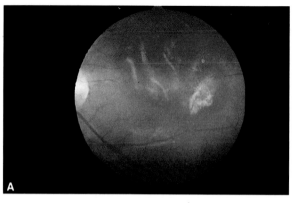

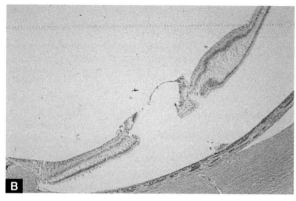

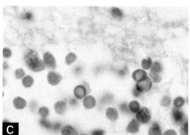

Fig. 3.7   Subacute Sclerosing Panencephalitis (SSPE). A The fundus of a patient who has SSPE shows acute retinitis in the region of the macula. **B** Histologic section shows necrosis of the central macula, resulting in hole formation. **C** Many intranuclear inclusion bodies are present in the inner nuclear layer. Patients presenting with SSPE frequently have ocular findings, mainly macular lesions and peripheral chorioretinal lesions. (**C**, modified from Nelson DA et al, 1970.)

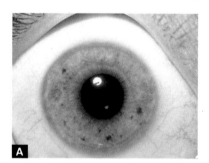

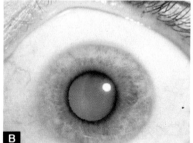

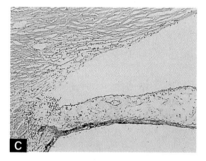

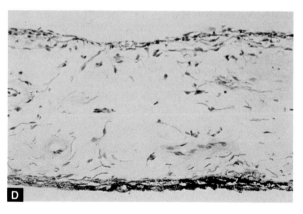

Fig. 3.8   Heterochromic Iridocyclitis (Fuchs). A The green iris of the normal uninvolved right eye is darker than in **B**, which shows the light blue iris in the involved left eye. Heterochromia, cataract (present in the left eye), and iris neovascularization are common in this condition. Loss of iris substance may become so severe that paradoxical heterochromia results in which only pigment epithelium remains in the involved eye, which then appears darker than the uninvolved eye. **C** Histologic section shows that diffuse trabeculitis and peripheral iritis are present. The inflammatory cells are mainly lymphocytes and plasma cells. **D** Marked atrophy of the iris and iris neovascularization are present. (**C, D**, case reported in Perry H et al, 1975.)

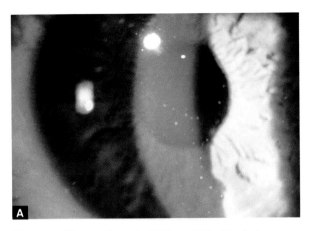 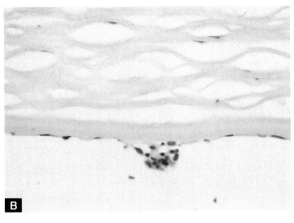

Fig. 3.9   Heterochromic Iridocyclitis (Fuchs).
A Slit lamp examination shows typical stellate keratic precipitates (KPs) which tend to change very little over long periods of time. **B** Histologic section shows that the KPs are composed of lymphocytes and histiocytes. (Case reported in Perry H et al, 1975.)

FIG. 3.10 SEQUELAE OF NONGRANULOMATOUS INFLAMMATION

Cornea
Endothelial cell loss
Corneal edema
Scarring
Band keratopathy
Vascularization
Anterior chamber and iris
Scarring
Iris neovascularization
Synechia, peripheral or posterior
Iris necrosis and atrophy
Lens and ciliary body
Cataract
Hyalinization of ciliary processes
Proliferation of ciliary epithelium
Cyclitic membrane

Vitreous and choroid
Posterior vitreous detachment
Cells in vitreous
Vitreous membranes
Atrophy and scarring of choroid
Retina and optic nerve
Perivasculitis of retina
Macular edema
Retinochoroidal scarring
Retinal detachment
Hyperplasia or atrophy of retinal
    pigment epithelium
Optic atrophy
Glaucoma
Secondary open-angle or closed-
    angle glaucoma may arise
    from numerous mechanisms

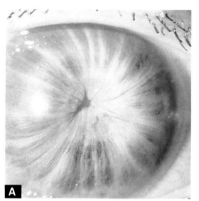

Fig. 3.11 Sequelae of Nongranulomatous Inflammation. A A membrane has grown across the pupil (occlusion of the pupil) and has adhered to the underlying lens, preventing the pupil from moving (seclusion of the pupil). **B** Aqueous in the posterior chamber has bowed the iris forward (iris bombé), resulting in peripheral anterior synechiae. **C** Histologic section of another case shows iris bombé, posterior synechiae of the iris to the anterior surface of the lens, a cyclitic membrane, and a retinal detachment. All are the result of long-standing chronic uveitis. (**A** and **B**, courtesy of Dr. GOH Naumann.)

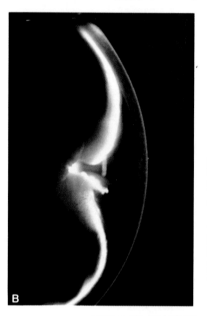

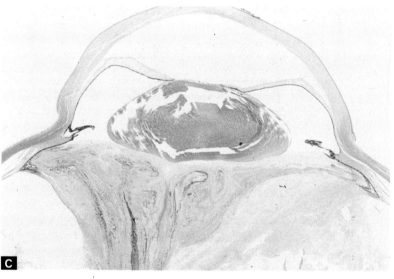

FIG. 3.12 END STAGE OF DIFFUSE OCULAR DISEASE

Atrophy without shrinkage (seen in chronic glaucoma)

Atrophy with shrinkage (atrophia bulbi; seen in chronic uveitis)

Atrophy with shrinkage and disorganization (phthisis bulbi; seen after purulent endophthalmitis)

Intraocular ossification (common with atrophia and phthisis bulbi)

Calcium deposition (may occur in many ocular structures)

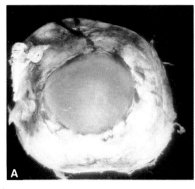 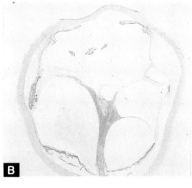 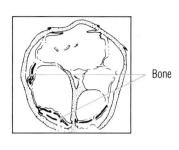

Bone

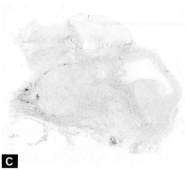

Fig. 3.13   End Stage of Diffuse Ocular Disease. A The enucleated eye shows the characteristic squared-off appearance of hypotony. The pull of the horizontal and vertical rectus muscles causes the soft, often shrunken, eye to appear squared-off or cuboidal. Clinically, this type of eye is called a phthisical eye or phthisis bulbi. However, histologically the eye is called atrophia bulbi. **B** Histologic section shows a small atrophic eye that is hypotonus, as evidenced by the ciliary body and choroidal detachments. Extensive formation of a rim of bone in the inner choroid can be seen. **C** In this histologic section, the globe is so disorganized that normal structures are unrecognizable. The condition is called phthisis bulbi. The eye is scarred completely after purulent endophthalmitis. (**C**, from *Ocular Pathology*, 2nd edn, by M Yanoff and BS Fine.)

Bibliography

de Abreu MT, et al: T-lymphocyte subsets in the aqueous humor and peripheral blood of patients with acute untreated uveitis. Am J Ophthalmol 98:62, 1984.

Kampik A, Patrinely JR, Green WR: Morphologic and clinical features of retrocorneal melanin pigmentation and pigmented pupillary membranes: review of 225 cases. Surv Ophthalmol 27:161, 1982.

Kijlstra A, Linssen A, Ockhuizen T: Association of GM allotypes with the occurrence of ankylosing spondylitis in HLA-B27-positive anterior uveitis. Am J Ophthalmol 98:732, 1984.

Nelson DA, et al: Retinal lesions in subacute sclerosing panencephalitis. Arch Ophthalmol 84:613, 1970.

O'Connor GR: Heterochromic iridocyclitis. Trans Ophthalmol Soc UK 104:219, 1985.

Pepose JS, et al: Immunocytologic localization of herpes simplex type 1 viral antigens in herpetic retinitis and encephalitis in an adult. Ophthalmology 92:160, 1985.

Perry H, Yanoff M, Scheie HG: Fuchs's heterochromic iridocyclitis. Arch Ophthalmol 93:337, 1975.

Pezzi PP, et al: Prognosis in Behçet's disease. Ann Ophthalmol 17:20, 1985.

Sheppard RD, Bornstein MB, Udem SA: Measles virus matrix protein synthesized in a subacute sclerosing panencephalitis cell line. Science 228:1219, 1985.

GRANULOMATOUS INFLAMMATION

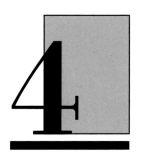

Granulomatous inflammation is a chronic, proliferative reaction characterized by a cellular infiltrate of epithelioid cells. Inflammatory giant cells, lymphocytes, plasma cells, polymorphonuclear leukocytes, and eosinophils also may be present. The identification of inflammation as granulomatous carries with it a high probability of finding a cause.

Often, the clinical information is helpful in determining the cause. For example, juvenile xanthogranuloma (JXG) occurs mainly in infants under 6 months of age, sarcoid in the third and fourth decades, and rheumatoid scleritis in the fifth and sixth decades. Race may be a factor in diagnosis as sarcoid occurs most commonly in blacks, and Vogt–Koyanagi–Harada disease occurs most often in orientals. A history of trauma should be determined. Following trauma, the most frequent complicating conditions include sympathetic uveitis, phacoanaphylactic endophthalmitis, and foreign body granulomas.

When nontraumatic inflammations are present, it is essential to differentiate whether the condition is infectious or noninfectious. The major infectious agents are viral entitites such as cytomegalic inclusion disease and herpes zoster; the main bacterial entities are tuberculosis, leprosy, syphilis, tularemia, and streptothrix or *Actinomyces* (a transitional organism between fungi and bacteria that now is classified as a bacterium). Major fungal entities are blastomycosis, cryptococcosis, coccidioidomycosis, aspergillosis, rhinosporidiosis, phycomycosis (mucormycosis or zygomycosis), candidiasis, histoplasmosis, and sporotrichosis. The most common parasitic entities found in granulomatous inflammation include toxoplasmosis, toxocariasis, trichinosis, loa loa, cysticercosis, hydatid cyst, and schistosomiasis.

A number of entities must be considered when it is determined that the inflammation is secondary neither to trauma nor to infection. The main considerations are sarcoidosis; granulomatous scleritis; chalazion; JXG; granulomatous reaction to Descemet's membrane; Chediak–Higashi syndrome; allergic granulomatosis; Vogt–Koyanagi–Harada syndrome; and familial, chronic, granulomatous disease of childhood.

Finally, as mentioned in Chapter 1, the pattern of inflammatory reaction may be quite helpful in diagnosing the particular type of granulomatous disease. If a *diffuse type* of reaction is found, the main causes are sympathetic uveitis, disseminated histoplasmosis and other fungal infections, lepromatous leprosy, JXG, Vogt–Koyanagi–Harada disease, cytomegalic inclusion disease, and toxoplasmosis. The epithelioid cells are distributed randomly against a background of lymphocytes and plasma cells. In the *discrete reaction*, the major causes are sarcoidosis, tuberculoid leprosy, and miliary tuberculosis. An accumulation of epithelioid cells forms nodules surrounded by a narrow rim of lymphocytes and some plasma cells. In the *zonal type* of reaction, the major causes are caseation tuberculosis, some fungal infections, rheumatoid scleritis, chalazion, phacoanaphylactic endophthalmitis, toxocariasis, and cysticercosis. A central nidus is surrounded by palisaded epithelioid cells that, in turn, usually are surrounded by lymphocytes and plasma cells.

Nongranulomatous inflammation is much more common than granulomatous inflammation. In nongranulomatous inflammation, however, the cause usually is not found, whereas in granulomatous inflammation the cause is found in a high percentage of cases. Both the history and the histological pattern of inflammation are the keys that help determine the cause.

FIG. 4.1 GRANULOMATOUS INFLAMMATION

Epithelioid cells necessary for diagnosis

Background of mononuclear cells

Giant cells often present

Reaction to persistent antigen

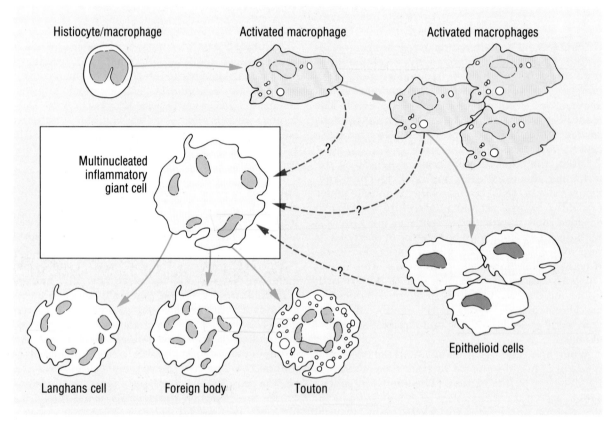

Fig. 4.2 Theoretical Origin of Epithelioid Cells and Inflammatory Giant Cells.

FIG. 4.3 GRANULOMATOUS INFLAMMATION CAUSED BY TRAUMA

Sympathetic uveitis

Follows penetrating ocular trauma

May develop 5 days to 20 + years after trauma (2 weeks is "safe period")

90% develop 2 weeks to 1 year after trauma (80% 3 weeks to 3 months)

Autoimmune reaction

Bilateral, diffuse, granulomatous uveitis

Histology

Diffuse, bilateral, granulomatous inflammation of uvea

Sparing of choriocapillaris

Pigment phagocytosis by epithelioid cells

Dalen–Fuchs nodules

Phacoanaphylactic endophthalmitis

Follows ocular trauma that results in a ruptured lens

Autoimmune reaction

Autosensitization to lens protein

Breakdown or reversal of central tolerance at T-lymphocyte level

Zonal granulomatous reaction

May be found concurrently in eyes that have sympathetic uveitis

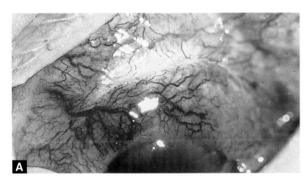

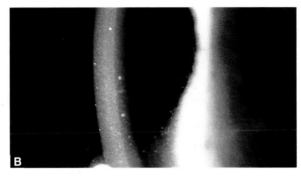

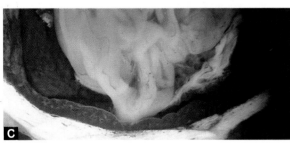

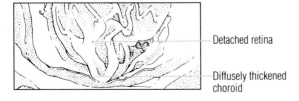

Detached retina

Diffusely thickened choroid

Fig. 4.4   Sympathetic Uveitis. A Blunt trauma resulted in rupture of the left globe and a hyphema. The patient developed photophobia in the uninjured right eye 7 weeks later. **B** Another patient shows mutton-fat, keratic precipitates. **C** Enucleated globe shows diffuse thickening of the choroid.

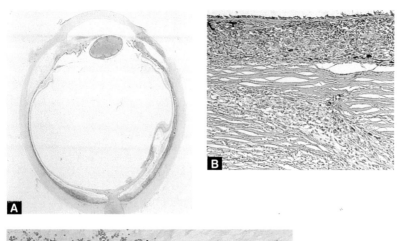

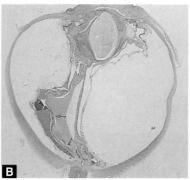

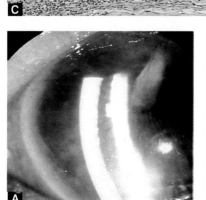

Fig. 4.5 Sympathetic Uveitis.
A Histologic section shows diffuse thickening of the choroid. **B** The choroid is thickened by a granulomatous, inflammatory reaction of the diffuse type. The pale areas represent epithelioid cell formation, and the dark areas consist mainly of lymphocytes. Sparing of the choriocapillaris and pigment phagocytosis by epithelioid cells are also seen. Note the granulomatous inflammatory involvement of a scleral canal in the lower right-hand corner of the picture. **C** A Dalen–Fuchs nodule, i.e., epithelioid cells between the pigment epithelium and Bruch's membrane, is present.

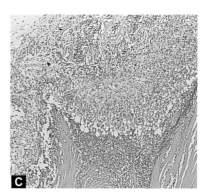

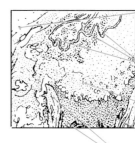

Lymphocytes, plasma cells, and fibrin

Ruptured lens capsule

Epithelioid cells

Polymorpho-nuclear leukocytes

Lens remnants

Fig. 4.6 Phacoanaphylactic Endophthalmitis. A The patient had an iridencleisis in 1971. The eye was injured by blunt trauma in an automobile accident in May 1973. In September 1973, signs and symptoms of an anterior uveitis developed. Note small, mutton-fat, keratic precipitates. The eye was enucleated in May 1974. **B** The enucleated globe shows iris in the subconjunctival tissue. The lens remnant, mainly nucleus, shows a zonal type of granulomatous reaction, consisting of surrounding epithelioid cells and giant cells, in turn surrounded by lymphocytes and plasma cells, in turn surrounded by granulation tissue. The lens capsule is ruptured posteriorly.
C Under increased magnification, the typical zonal pattern is seen around the remnant of lens nucleus. (**B**, PAS.)

FIG. 4.7 GRANULOMATOUS INFLAMMATION CAUSED BY INFECTIONS

Viral
Cytomegalic inclusion disease
Herpes zoster (shingles)
Bacterial
Tuberculosis
Leprosy
Syphilis
Tularemia
Streptothrix (*Actinomyces*)

Fungal
Blastomycosis
Cryptococcosis
Coccidioidomycosis
Rhinosporidiosis
Phycomycosis (mucormycosis,
   zygomycosis)
Candidiasis
Histoplasmosis
Sporotrichosis

Parasitic
Toxoplasmosis (Protozoa)
Toxocariasis (Nematoda)
Trichinosis (Nematoda)
Loa loa (Nematoda)
Cysticercosis (Cestoidea)
Hydatid cyst (Cestoidea)
Schistosomiasis (Trematoda)

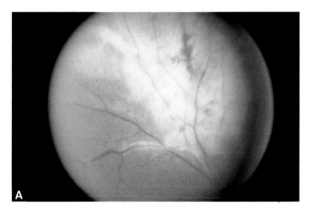

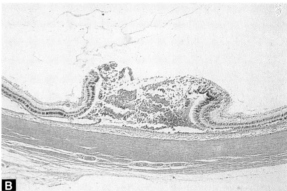

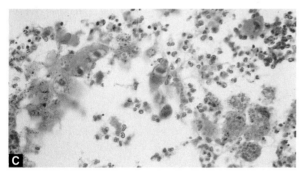

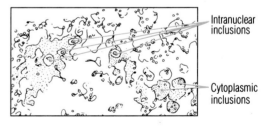

Intranuclear inclusions

Cytoplasmic inclusions

Fig. 4.8 Cytomegalic Inclusion Disease. A The fundus picture shows the characteristic hemorrhagic exudation along the retinal vessels. **B** Histologic section shows the relatively normal retina sharply demarcated from the area of coagulative retinal necrosis, secondary to the infection. The choroid shows a secondary, mild, diffuse, granulomatous inflammation. **C** Increased magnification shows typical, eosinophilic, intranuclear inclusion bodies and small, round, basophilic, cytoplasmic inclusion bodies. (**A**, courtesy Dr. S.H. Sinclair; case shown in **B** and **C** presented by Dr. Daniel Toussaint at Verhoeff Society Meeting, 1976.)

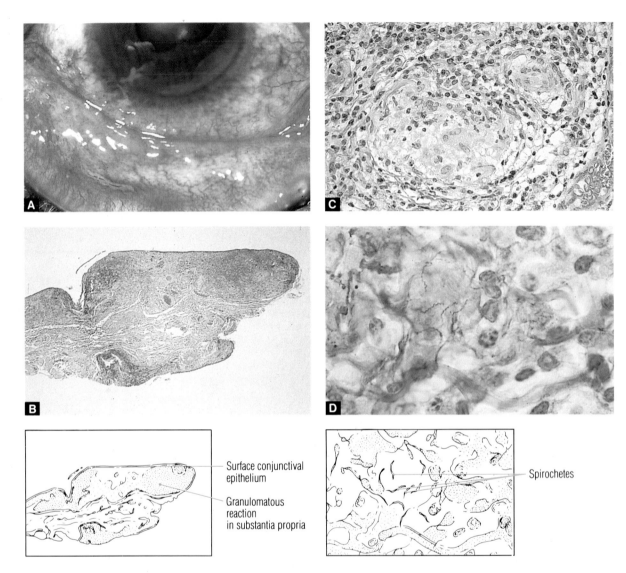

Fig. 4.9 Syphilis. A Small, round, translucent nodules are seen in the conjunctiva of the inferior fornix. **B** The biopsied nodules show numerous granulomas under the conjunctival epithelium. **C** Increased magnification reveals epithelioid cells within the inflammatory nodules. **D** A special stain demonstrates spirochetes within the inflammatory infiltrate.(**D**, Dieterla; case reported in Spektor FE, et al:Ophthalmology 88:863, 1981.)

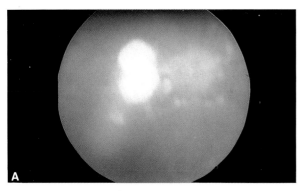

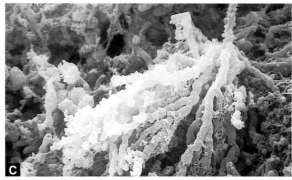

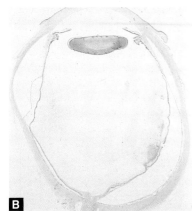

Fig. 4.10 Fungal Endophthalmitis. A Immunosuppressed patient developed endophthalmitis. Note the "snowball" opacities in the vitreous just around the optic nerve head. *Candida albicans* was cultured from the blood. **B** Another patient developed decreased vision in his right eye, followed by renal failure 2 months after a kidney transplant. He died 1 month later. The histologic section shows microabscesses within the vitreous body, characteristic of fungal infection (bacterial infection causes a diffuse vitreous abscess). **C** Scanning electron microscopy demonstrates septate branching *Aspergillus* hyphae. (**C**, courtesy of Dr. R.C. Eagle, Jr, from *Ocular Pathology*, 2nd edn, by M Yanoff and BS Fine.)

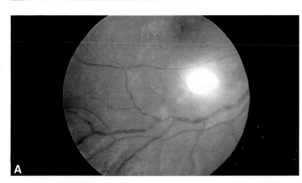

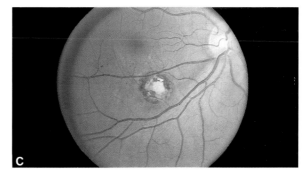

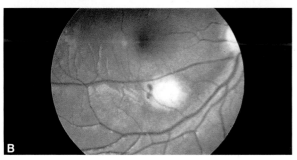

Fig. 4.11 Toxoplasmosis. A A 12-year-old girl developed an acute endophthalmitis in her right eye in May 1970. The tiny, brown balls on the retinal venules probably represent small granulomas. **B** Early pigmentation is present 7 years later. **C** Twelve years later, in 1982, increased pigmentation now makes the lesion appear like a typical toxoplasmosis lesion. (From *Ocular Pathology*, 2nd edn, by M Yanoff and BS Fine.)

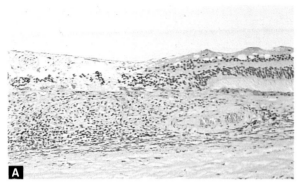

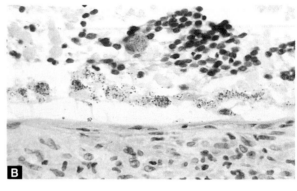

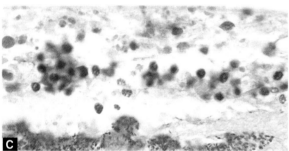

Fig. 4.12 **Toxoplasmosis.** **A** Histologic section showing an acute, coagulative retinal necrosis, whereas the choroid shows a secondary, diffuse, granulomatous inflammation. **B** A toxoplasmic cyst is present in the retina. Note the tiny nuclei within the cyst. **C** In another section, free forms of the protozoa are present in the necrotic retina. The tiny nuclei are eccentrically placed and the opposite end of the cytoplasm tends to taper.

FIG. 4.13 NONTRAUMATIC, NONINFECTIOUS TYPES OF GRANULOMATOUS INFLAMMATION

Sarcoidosis

Granulomatous scleritis

Chalazion

Juvenile xanthogranuloma (JXG)

Granulomatous reaction to Descemet's membrane

Chediak–Higashi syndrome

Vogt–Koyanagi–Harada syndrome

Familial chronic granulomatous disease of childhood

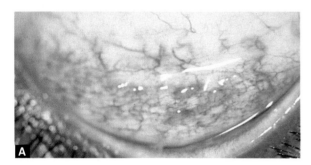

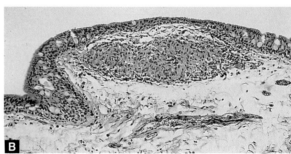

Fig. 4.14 **Sarcoidosis.** **A** The patient shows numerous, small, round, translucent cysts in the conjunctival fornix. **B** A conjunctival biopsy reveals a discrete granuloma, composed of epithelioid cells, and surrounded by a rim of lymphocytes and plasma cells. Such granulomas may be found histologically even if no conjunctival nodules are noted clinically.

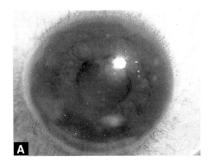

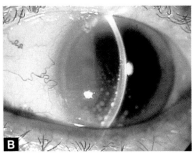

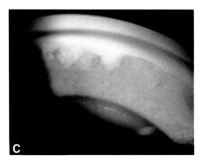

Fig. 4.15 Sarcoidosis. A The iris is involved in the granulomatous process and shows numerous, large granulomas. **B** Slit lamp view shows numerous mutton-fat keratic precipitates. **C** Granulomas and peripheral anterior synechiae are noted in the angle of the anterior chamber.

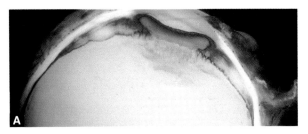

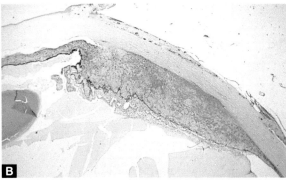

Fig. 4.16 Sarcoidosis. A The enucleated globe shows an infiltrate in the ciliary body. **B** The infiltrate consists of a discrete, granulomatous inflammation.

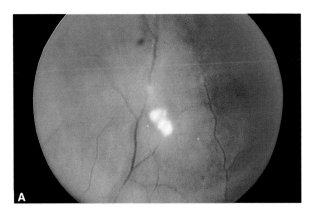

Fig. 4.17 Sarcoidosis. A White, cellular masses ("balls") are seen in the vitreous compartment on the surface of the retina inferiorly along with early "candle wax drippings". **B** White balls are caused by accumulations of epithelioid cells in the vitreous and candle wax drippings by perivascular, granulomatous infiltration in the retina. Candle wax drippings are often an ominous sign, because they may be associated with central nervous system sarcoidosis. Note Dalen–Fuchs nodule on the right. (**B**, case reported in Gass JDM, Olsen CL: Arch Ophthalmol 94:945, 1976.)

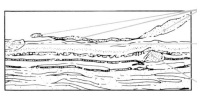

Epithelioid cells in vitreous

Perivascular granulomatous retinal inflammation

Dalen–Fuchs nodule

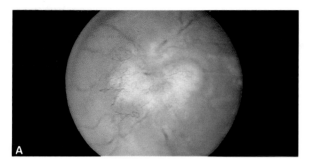

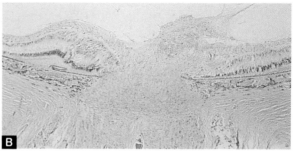

Fig. 4.18 Sarcoidosis. A The optic nerve is involved in a mass of granulomas. **B** Histologic section of another patient shows granulomatous inflammation in the anterior portion of the optic nerve. (**A**, courtesy of Dr. A.J. Brucker; **B**, this case reported in Gass JDM, Olsen CL: Trans Am Acad Ophthalmol Otolaryngol 77:739, 1973.)

Bibliography

Chan C-C, et al: Granulomas in sympathetic ophthalmia and sarcoidosis. Arch Ophthalmol 103:198, 1985.

Chan C-C, et al: Anti-retinal auto-antibodies in Vogt–Koyanagi–Harada syndrome, Behçet's disease, and sympathetic ophthalmia. Ophthalmology 92:1025, 1985.

Chandler FW, et al: Zygomycosis. Report of four cases with formation of chlamydoconidia in tissue. Am J Clin Pathol 84:99, 1985.

Fung JC, et al: Serologic diagnosis of toxoplasmosis with emphasis on the detection of toxoplasma-specific immunoglobin M antibodies. Am J Clin Pathol 83:196, 1985.

Gass JDM, Olsen CL: Sarcoidosis with optic nerve and retinal involvement. Arch Ophthalmol 94:945, 1976.

Khalil M, Lindley S, Matouk E: Tuberculosis of the orbit. Ophthalmology 92:1624, 1985.

Kleiner RC, Raber IM, Passero FC: Scleritis, pericarditis, and aortic insufficiency in a patient with rheumatoid arthritis. Ophthalmol 91:941, 1984.

Kruger-Lite E, et al: Intraocular cysticercosis. Am J Ophthalmol 99:252, 1985.

Marak GE, Font RL, Alepa FP: Immunopathogenicity of lens crystallins in the production of experimental lens-induced granulomatous endophthalmitis. Ophthalmic Res 10:33, 1978.

McDonnell PJ, et al: Ocular involvement in patients with fungal infections. Ophthalmology 92:706, 1985.

Nichols CW, et al: Conjunctival biopsy as an aid in evaluation of the patient with suspected sarcoidosis. Ophthalmology 87:287, 1980.

Rao NA, Shizhao X, Font RL: Sympathetic Ophthalmia: an immunohistochemical study of epithelioid and giant cells. Ophthalmology 92:1160, 1985.

Rodrigues MM, et al: Unilateral cytomegalovirus retinochoroiditis and bilateral cytoid bodies in a bisexual man with acquired immunodeficiency syndrome. Ophthalmology 90:1577, 1983.

Shields JA: Ocular toxocariasis. A review. Surv Ophthalmol 28:361, 1984.

Spaide R, et al: Ocular findings in leprosy in the United States. Am J Ophthalmol 100:411, 1985.

Spektor FE, Eagle RC Jr, Nichols CW: Granulomatous conjunctivitis secondary to *Treponema pallidum*. Ophthalmology 88:863,1981.

SURGICAL AND NONSURGICAL TRAUMA 5

COMPLICATIONS OF INTRAOCULAR SURGERY

Complications of intraocular surgery may occur immediately, during the postoperative period, or may be delayed. The "immediate" period is from the time the decision is made to perform surgery until the patient leaves the operating room. The postoperative period extends from the time the patient leaves the operating room until about 3 months after surgery. The delayed period occurs after the third month following surgery. Cataract surgery will be used as the prototype for intraocular surgery. Many complications occur because appropriate planning and techniques are not used. It is important to make the correct diagnosis before the surgery is decided. There are numerous examples of uveal melanomas and ocular retinoblastomas being discovered after cataracts have been removed, the cataracts having formed secondary to the tumors. At the time of surgery, the technique must be meticulous. A perfectly performed procedure can end in a disaster simply because of inadequate anesthesia. Even when everything goes well, however, complications may occur. Some of the common and important types of complications will be illustrated.

COMPLICATIONS OF NONSURGICAL TRAUMA

Broadly speaking, nonsurgical trauma can be divided into two types: trauma following a contusion; and trauma following penetrating and perforating ocular injuries. A contusion results from an external (direct or indirect) force on the eye. The most common contusive injury is one that results from direct, blunt trauma to the eye. The contusion is the injury that results from the force propagated throughout the eye (i.e., the concussive force). Every part of the eye can be affected. An injury may be so severe that a tissue or structure of the eye is partially cut or torn, resulting in a penetrating or perforating injury. When this occurs, aside from the effects of contusion, the effects of the torn tissue must be considered. Rupture of the globe usually occurs at its thinnest parts: the limbus; the sclera, just posterior to the insertion of the rectus muscles; or just adjacent to the optic nerve. At the time of perforation, sterile or contaminated objects may be introduced to the interior of the eye and their added effects must also be considered.

In addition to penetrating and perforating injuries, other types of injuries may involve the eye. Chemicals may be splashed into the eye. The eyes may be involved in burns or radiation-induced injuries. Injuries to other parts of the body may have ocular effects, e.g., traumatic carotid-carvernous fistula. Examples of some of the common important types of nonsurgical trauma will be illustrated.

Fig. 5.1 IMMEDIATE COMPLICATIONS OF INTRAOCULAR SURGERY

Misdiagnosis
Cataract may be secondary to inflammation or neoplasm
Retinal detachment may be secondary to inflammation or neoplasm

Faulty surgical technique
Inadequate facial or retrobulbar anesthesia
Retrobulbar hemorrhage
Misplacement of incision or of sutures
Stripping of Descemet's membrane
Iridodialysis

Vitreous loss
Expulsive choroidal hemorrhage

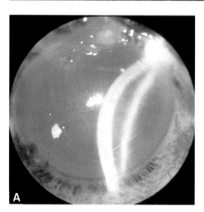

Fig. 5.2 Stripping of Descemet's Membrane. A Descemet's membrane was stripped over a large area during filtration surgery. The edge of Descemet's membrane, free in the anterior chamber, can be seen to the right of the slit lamp corneal reflex. **B** The gross specimen shows the stripped Descemet's membrane between the iris and the cornea. **C** Histology demonstrates the region of filtration. Descemet's membrane can be seen in the anterior chamber between the iris and the cornea. (Case reported in Kozart DM, Eagle RC Jr:Ophthalmic Surg 12:420, 1981.)

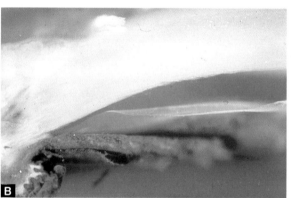

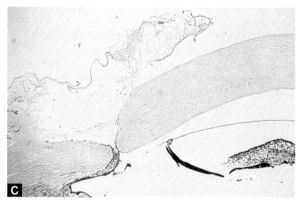

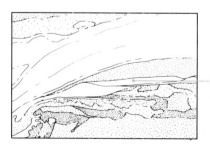

Stripped Descemet's membrane

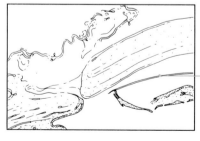

Stripped Descemet's membrane

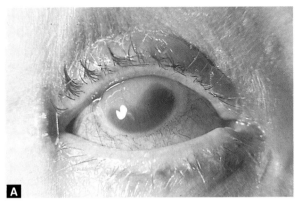

A

Fig. 5.3 Expulsive Choroidal Hemorrhage. A A large hyphema is present in the anterior chamber. The patient had an expulsive choroidal hemorrhage during surgery. **B** Histologic section shows hemorrhage in the choroid and subretinal space. The retina is in the corneoscleral wound. (**A**, courtesy of Dr. HG Scheie.)

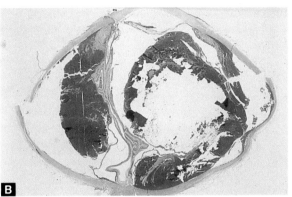

B

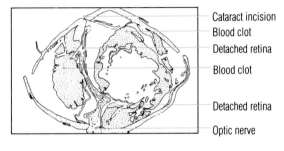

Cataract incision
Blood clot
Detached retina
Blood clot

Detached retina
Optic nerve

Fig. 5.4 POSTOPERATIVE COMPLICATIONS OF INTRAOCULAR SURGERY

Flat chamber
Faulty wound closure
Choroidal detachment
Aphakic or pseudophakic
    glaucoma
Choroidal hemorrhage
Iris incarceration or prolapse
Fistulization of cataract wound
Poor wound healing
Striate keratopathy
Hyphema

Corneal edema
Secondary to increased
    intraocular pressure
Secondary to corneal endothelial
    damage
Secondary to adherent vitreous
    or iris
Secondary to splitting off of
    Descemet's membrane
Aggravation of Fuchs combined
    dystrophy
Subretinal hemorrhage
Retinal detachment
**Inflammation (may be
    infectious, usually bacteria,
    or noninfectious)**

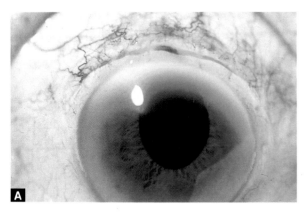

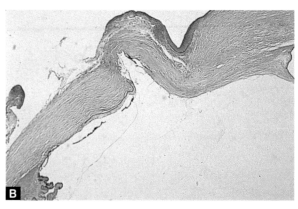

Fig. 5.5 Iris in the Wound. A Two weeks postoperatively, the iris has prolapsed through the wound and presents subconjunctivally at the 12- o'clock position. **B** In this case, the iris has become incarcerated within the wound, causing the internal portion of the wound to gape.

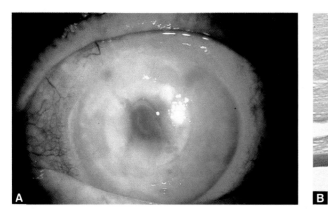

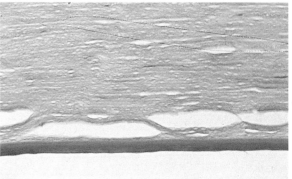

Fig. 5.6 Corneal Edema. A Corneal edema has led to bullous keratopathy in this patient with an iris clip intraocular lens. **B** No endothelium is present on Descemet's membrane. The normally seen artifactious clefts in the cornea are largely obliterated by edema fluid in the corneal stroma. (**A**, courtesy of Dr. IM Raber.)

Fig. 5.7 DELAYED COMPLICATIONS OF INTRAOCULAR SURGERY		
Corneal edema	**Glaucoma**	**Inflammation**
Elschnig's pearls	Peripheral anterior synechiae	Infectious—usually fungal or *Staphylococcus epidermidis*
Soemmerring ring cataract	Posterior synechiae	Uveitis
Retinal detachment	Epithelial downgrowth (or cyst)	Sympathetic uveitis
	Stromal overgrowth	Phacoanaphylactic endophthalmitis
	Endothelial overgrowth	**Cystoid macular edema**
		Atrophia or phthisis bulbi

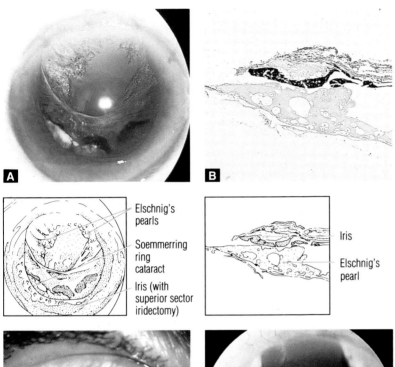

Fig. 5.8 Elschnig's Pearls and Soemmerring Ring Cataract.
A Elschnig's pearls are seen as translucent, tiny spheres in the superior, peripheral pupillary space. Cortical remnants, in the form of a Soemmerring ring cataract, are noted from six to eight o'clock. **B** Pearls are caused by aberrant attempts by the lens cells to form new lens "fibers", often in close association with a Soemmerring ring cataract. A Soemmerring ring cataract is caused by cortical material being trapped in the equatorial portion of the lens in a doughnut configuration. (**A**, from *Ocular Pathology*, 2nd edn, by M Yanoff and BS Fine.)

Elschnig's pearls

Soemmerring ring cataract

Iris (with superior sector iridectomy)

Iris

Elschnig's pearl

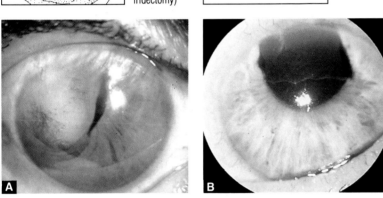

Corneal scar

Epithelial downgrowth

Fig. 5.9 Epithelial Ingrowth. A Implantation of epithelium on the iris at the time of surgery has resulted in the formation of a large, epithelial cyst that obstructs most of the pupil. The milky material within the cyst consists of desquamated epithelial cells. **B** In another case, the epithelium has grown into the eye through the cataract incision and is developing as a downgrowth on the back of the superior one-third of the cornea and onto the superior iris. The line of transition between epithelium and endothelium is seen clearly on the posterior cornea as a horizontal line.
C Epithelium is present over the posterior surface of the cornea, within the angle, over the iris, and extending posteriorly onto the vitreous.
(**B**, case reported in Yanoff M:Trans Am Ophthalmol Soc 73:571, 1975; from *Ocular Pathology*, 2nd edn, by M Yanoff and BS Fine.)

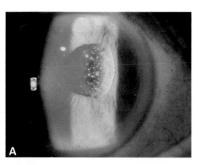

Fig. 5.10   Intraocular Lens Inflammation. A Large, pigmented precipitates are present on the anterior and posterior surface of the lens. Entrapment of the posterior chamber lens has taken place on the right-hand side of the pupil. **B** This anterior chamber lens was removed because of the uveitis, glaucoma, hyphema (UGH) syndrome. The lens is covered with precipitates. **C** Increased magnification shows many histiocytes and multinucleated giant cells on the lens surface. (**B, C,** courtesy of Dr. R.C. Eagle, Jr.)

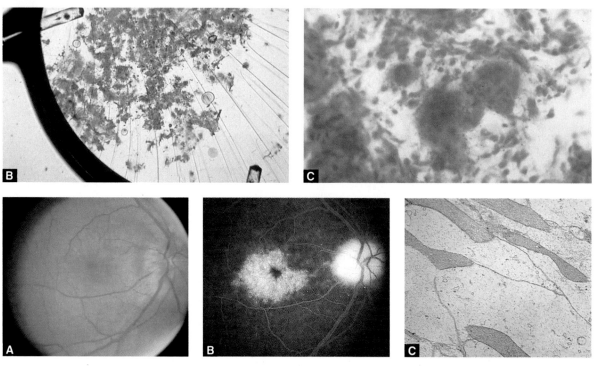

Fig. 5.11   Cystoid Macular Edema. After extracapsular cataract extraction and posterior chamber lens implantation, the patient initially did well. Then however, vision decreased. **A** Examination of the fundus showed cystoid macular edema. **B** The characteristic fluorescein appearance is present. The patient's vision was decreased to 20/300. No treatment was given. Nine months later the vision spontaneously returned to 20/20. **C** Electron microscopy of another case shows intracytoplasmic accumulation of fluid within Müller cells. Early, the fluid in cystoid macular edema is intracytoplasmic and the condition is reversible. Further accumulation of fluid causes the cell membranes to break, the fluid collects extracellularly, and presumably the condition is irreversible. (**C,** modified from Yanoff M, et al:Surv Ophthalmol 28 [Suppl]:505, 1984.)

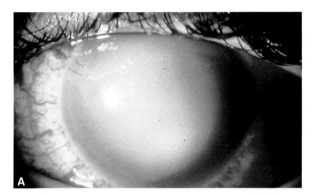

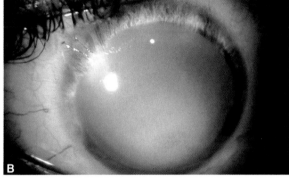

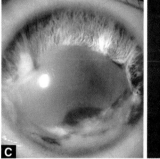
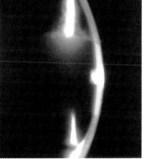

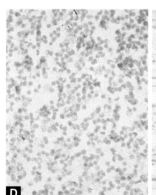
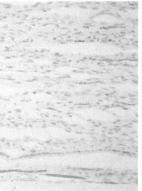

Fig. 5.13 Hyphema. A The patient sustained a blunt trauma that resulted in a total hyphema. One month later, blood staining has occurred. **B** Three months after the initial injury, the hyphema is starting to clear peripherally. **C** One year after the trauma, most of the cornea is cleared. **D** Histological sections of a case of corneal blood staining shows intact red blood cells in the anterior chamber on the left side. The right side, taken at the same magnification, shows the cornea in the same case; both are stained for iron. The red blood cells in the cornea have broken up into hemoglobin particles and do not stain for iron. The only positive staining for iron is within the cytoplasm of corneal keratocytes. (**D**, left and right, Perl's stain.)

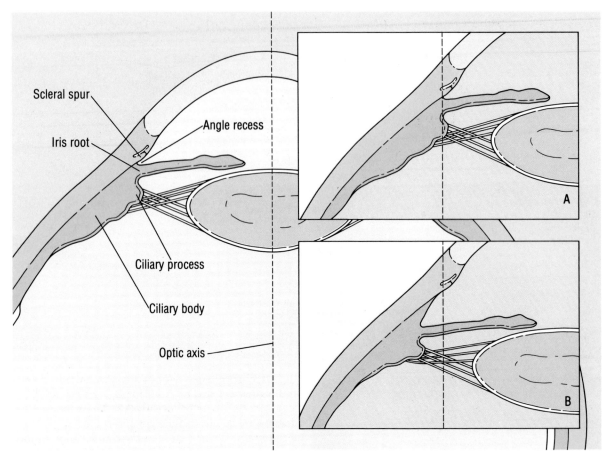

Fig. 5.14 Angle recession. A A line drawn parallel to the optic axis in a normal eye passes through the scleral spur, the angle recess, the iris root, and the most anterior portion of the ciliary processes. The ciliary body has a wedge shape, i.e., is pointed at its posterior portion but straight-sided anteriorly. **B** In an eye that has an angle recession (also called postcontusion deformity of the anterior chamber angle), the line parallel to the optic axis that passes through the scleral spur will pass anterior to the angle recess, the iris root, and the most anterior portion of the ciliary body. The ciliary body is fusiform, i.e., pointed posteriorly and anteriorly. (In a fetal or neonatal eye, the line parallel to the optic axis that passes through the scleral spur will pass posterior to the angle recess, iris root, and the most anterior portion of the ciliary body and the ciliary body has a normal wedge shape.)

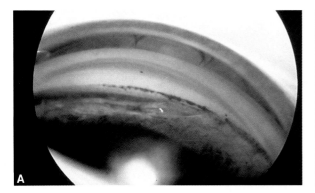

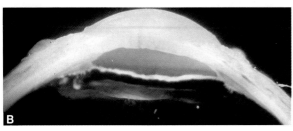

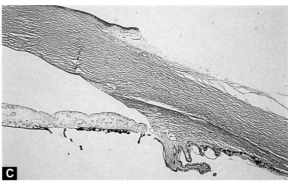

Fig. 5.15 Angle Recession. A The angle of the anterior chamber in an eye of a patient who had sustained a blunt trauma is of normal depth over the right side of the figure except for peripheral anterior synechiae but is markedly deepened and recessed over the left side. **B** A gross specimen from another case shows the deepened anterior chamber and recessed angle. The fusiform (pointed at both ends) shape of the ciliary body (most clearly seen on the right) is characteristic of angle recession. **C** The ciliary body inserts into the scleral spur normally. The oblique and circular muscles of the ciliary body have atrophied, following a laceration into the anterior face of the ciliary body, and the resulting scar tissue has contracted, pulling the angle recess, iris root, and ciliary processes posteriorly. The anterior wedge shape of the ciliary body has been lost. The entire process results in a fusiform shape of the ciliary body. A number of mechanisms such as trabecular damage and late scarring, peripheral anterior synechiae, and endothelialization of an open angle, can lead to secondary glaucoma that would result in optic nerve damage.

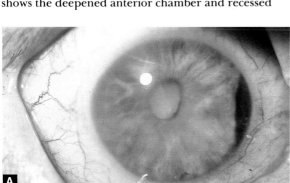

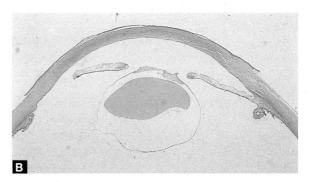

Fig. 5.16 Iridodialysis. A The patient sustained blunt trauma that resulted in an iridodialysis. Over the next few months he developed a mature cataract. The NLP eye was enucleated. **B** Histological section shows that the liquified cortex has completely leaked out from the lens during tissue processing; all that remains is the nucleus, surrounded by a clear area where the cortex had been, surrounded by the lens capsule. Note the anterior subcapsular cataract. The iridodialysis is seen on the left. In addition, the fusiform shape of the ciliary body, best seen on the right, is the clue that an angle recession is present (**A** from *Ocular Pathology*, 2nd edn, by M Yanoff and BS Fine; **B**, PAS.)

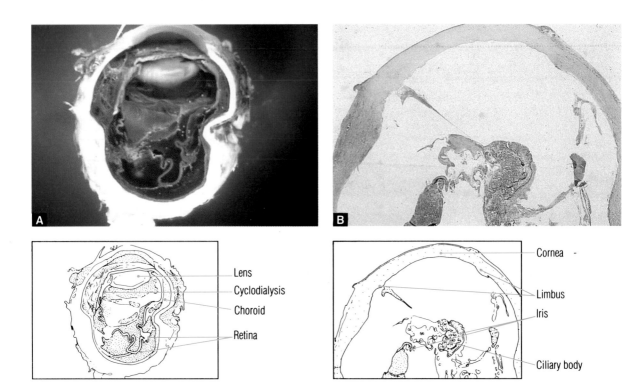

Lens
Cyclodialysis
Choroid

Retina

Cornea
Limbus
Iris

Ciliary body

Fig. 5.17 Cyclodialysis. A The gross eye shows the ciliary body attached to the scleral spur on the right side. The entire ciliary body on the left side, however, is avulsed from the scleral spur, resulting in a cyclodialysis. **B** Histologic section from another case shows the ciliary body and iris in the center of the eye, avulsed from the scleral spur 360° degrees.

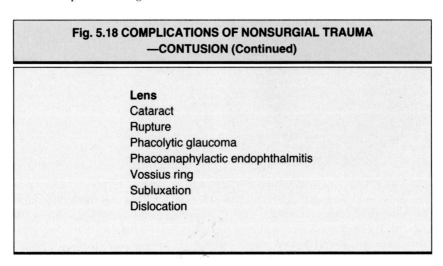

Fig. 5.18 COMPLICATIONS OF NONSURGIAL TRAUMA —CONTUSION (Continued)

Lens
Cataract
Rupture
Phacolytic glaucoma
Phacoanaphylactic endophthalmitis
Vossius ring
Subluxation
Dislocation

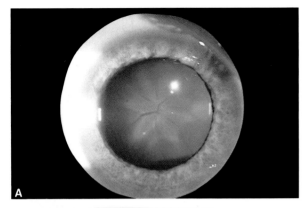

Fig. 5.19 Traumatic Cataract. A The patient had blunt trauma from years past. A typical, petal-shaped cataract has developed. This may develop in the cortex, under the anterior capsule, or under the posterior capsule. In this case, the cataract is present in both the anterior and posterior cortex. **B** Histologic section of another petal-shaped traumatic cataract shows anterior and posterior cortical degeneration in the form of narrow bands (seen under increased magnification in **C** and **D**). The bands are responsible for the "petals" seen clinically.

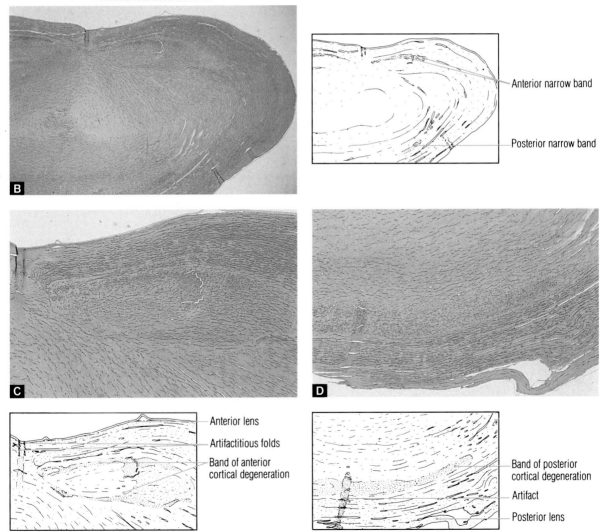

Anterior narrow band

Posterior narrow band

Anterior lens

Artifactitious folds

Band of anterior cortical degeneration

Band of posterior cortical degeneration

Artifact

Posterior lens

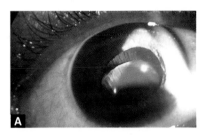

Fig. 5.20 Lens Subluxation and Disclocation. A The lens is subluxed inferiorly so that the zonular fibers are easily noted in the superior pupil. When a lens is subluxated, it is still in the posterior chamber but not in its normal position. **B** The lens is dislocated into the anterior chamber. Pupillary block has resulted in peripheral anterior syechiae and closed-angle glaucoma (a similar case is shown histologically in **C**). (**A**, from *Ocular Pathology*, 2nd edn, by M Yanoff and BS Fine.)

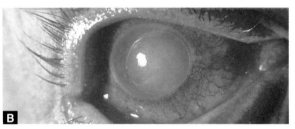

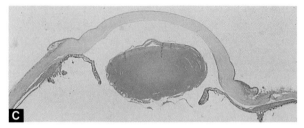

Fig. 5.21 COMPLICATIONS OF NONSURGICAL TRAUMA—CONTUSION (Continued)

Ciliary body and choroid

Hemorrhage	Cyclitic membrane	Chorioretinopathy
Inflammation	Choroidal rupture	

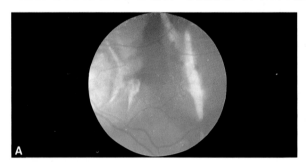

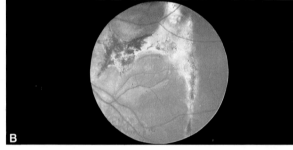

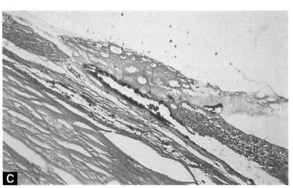

Fig. 5.22 Chroidal Rupture. A The patient sustained a blunt trauma that resulted in choroidal ruptures in the posterior pole and in subneural retinal hemorrhages. The optic nerve head is on the left in this eye. **B** One year later, considerable scarring has taken place. These cases must be watched closely for the occurrence of subneural retinal neovascularization that may occur at the edge of the healed rupture. **C** Histologic section of another case shows rupture of the choroid following blunt trauma. (**C**, courtesy of Dr. WR Green, reported in Aguilar JP and Green WR: Retina 4:269, 1984.)

Fig. 5.23 COMPLICATIONS OF NONSURGICAL TRAUMA—CONTUSION (Continued)

Vitreous		
Inflammation	Hemorrhage	Cholesterolosis

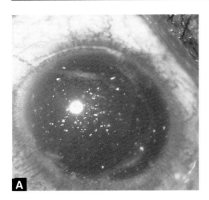

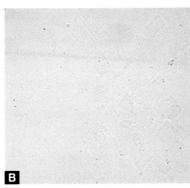

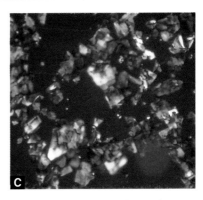

Fig. 5.24   Cholesterolosis. A A traumatic hyphema has absorbed but cholesterol remains in the anterior chamber. **B** An anterior chamber aspirate of another case shows cholesterol crystals. **C** The cholesterol crystals are birefringent to polarized light. (**B**, unstained **C**, unstained and polarized.)

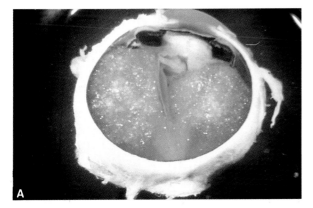

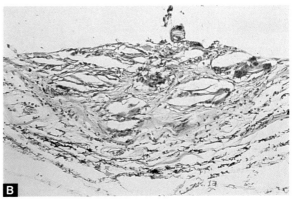

Fig. 5.25   Cholesterolosis. A The subneural retinal space is filled with an exudate containing many cholesterol crystals. Cholesterol often settles out following vitreous or subneural retinal hemorrhages. **B** The cholesterol may be seen free as, in **A** and in Fig. 5.24, or the clefts may appear as empty spaces, surrounded by foreign body giant cells. The cholesterol itself is dissolved out by processing of the tissue and only the space remains where the cleft had been. (**B**, from *Ocular Pathology*, 2nd edn, by M Yanoff and BS Fine.)

Fig. 5.26 COMPLICATIONS OF NONSURGICAL TRAUMA —CONTUSION (Continued)

Retina
Commotio retinae
 (Berlin's edema)
Hemorrhages
Tears
Optic nerve
Partial or complete avulsion
Hemorrhage
Optic disc edema

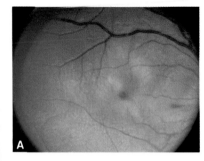
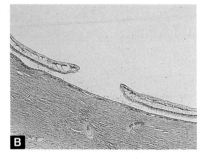

Fig. 5.27 Commotio Retinae. (Berlin's Edema) A The posterior pole is milky and opaque because of damage in the form of vacuolization and degeneration of the inner portion of the photoreceptor and outer nuclear layers. **B** Following commotio retinae, some cases will heal with pigmentation. In other cases, fluid will enter the macular retinal region and cause microcystoid degeneration. Hole formation ultimately may result as noted here.

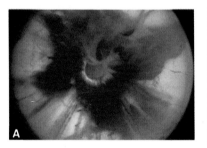

Fig. 5.28 Avulsion of the Optic Nerve. A Following trauma, the optic nerve has been avulsed. Note the hole opening into the orbit where the optic nerve had been. **B** The scleral optic nerve canal is not filled with optic nerve but contains retina. (**A**, case courtesy of Dr. ME Smith.)

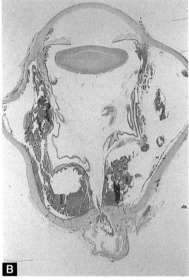

Fig. 5.29 COMPLICATIONS OF NONSURGICAL TRAUMA —CONTUSION (Continued)

Glaucoma
Closed angle
Secondary to repair
Organization of hemorrhage
 and exudate
Endothelialization
Iris neovascularization
Open angle
Cells and debris
Angle recession
Trabecular damage

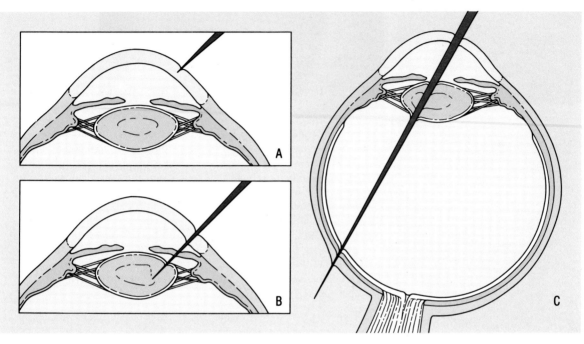

Fig. 5.30 PENETRATION AND PERFORATION OF THE GLOBE—DEFINITIONS

Penetration—into but not through   Perforation—into and through

Fig. 5.31   Penetration and Perforation of the Globe.
A The arrow shows a penetrating wound of the cornea. **B** The arrow shows a perforating wound of the cornea and iris and a penetrating wound of the lens and globe. **C** The arrow shows a perforating wound of the cornea, lens, retina, choroid, sclera, and globe.

Fig 5.32 PENETRATION AND PERFORATION OF THE GLOBE—SIGNS

Decreased visual acuity
Hypotony
Shallow anterior chamber
  (anterior perforation)
Deep anterior chamber
  (posterior perforation)
Pupillary alteration
Blood in vitreous
Obvious ocular laceration

Fig. 5.33 PENETRATION AND PERFORATION OF THE GLOBE—EFFECTS

Corneal and scleral rupture
Prolapse or loss of intraocular contents
Epithelial downgrowth
Stromal overgrowth
Intraocular infection
Intraocular foreign body
Effects of contusion

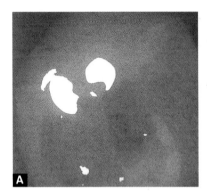

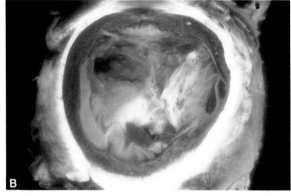

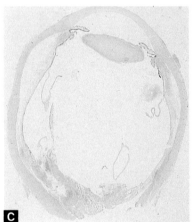

Fig. 5.34 Rupture of the Globe. A A patient had a gunshot injury to the globe. X-ray examination shows multiple metallic foreign bodies within the globe. The eye was enucleated. **B**. The gross specimen shows disorganization, hemorrhage, and retinal detachment. A rupture of the choroid and retina can be seen at the 4-o'clock position at the site of an exit wound. In enucleating the hypotonus globe the surgeon cut across the sclera, leaving the optic nerve head with its surrounding sclera, choroid, and retina in the orbit. Obviously, because of uveal tissue left in the orbit, the patient is a candidate for sympathetic uveitis. **C** Histologic section shows the detached retina and the "button-hole" of the posterior segment. Note an opaque, black foreign body on the internal surface of the ciliary body on the right side.

Fig. 5.35 INTRAOCULAR FOREIGN BODIES
Inorganic Relatively inert—gold, silver, platinum, aluminum, and glass Relatively active—iron and copper **Organic** Vegetable matter—often contaminated with opportunistic fungi Cilium

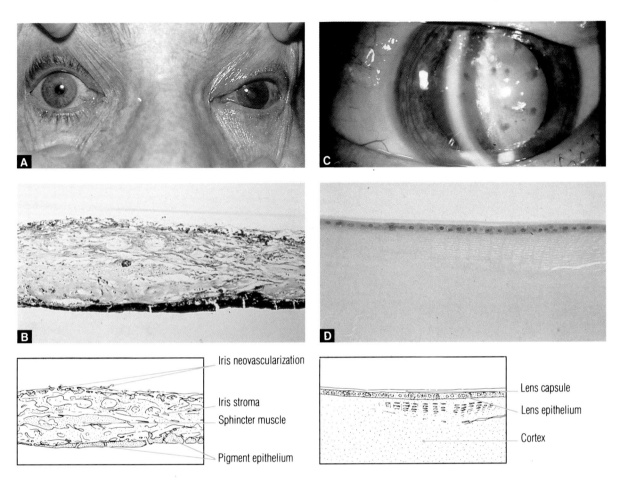

Iris neovascularization

Iris stroma

Sphincter muscle

Pigment epithelium

Lens capsule

Lens epithelium

Cortex

Fig. 5.36 Siderosis Bulbi. A The patient has an intraocular iron foreign body in his left eye. Pigmentation has caused the left iris to become dark. **B** A Special stain that demonstrates iron by a blue color shows the presence of iron diffusely in the stroma of the iris. Iron was also present in the anterior layer of the iris pigment epithelium. Note the presence of iris neovascularization. **C** The patient had a long-standing hemorrhage in the eye. Iron deposition in the lens has caused hemosiderosis lentis. Hemosiderosis and siderosis are indistinguishable histologically. **D** Iron, as noted by the blue color, is deposited in the lens epithelium and not in the lens capsule or cortex (**A**, from *Ocular Pathology*, 2nd edn, by M Yanoff and BS Fine, **B**, Perl's stain; **D**, Perl's stain.)

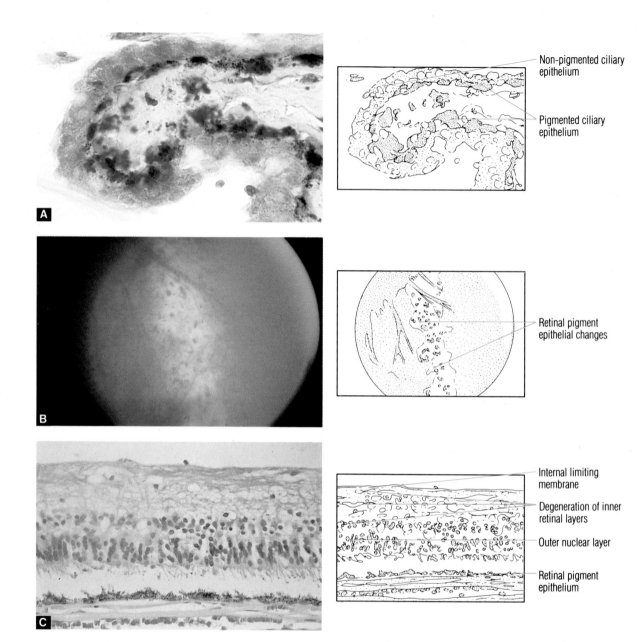

Fig. 5.37 Siderosis and Hemosiderosis Bulbi. In both conditions, iron may be deposited in neuroepithelial and lens epithelial structures such as iris pigment epithelium, lens epithelium, corneal epithelium, and ciliary epithelium (**A**), and pigment epithelium of the retina. Iron also may be deposited in the iris stroma, the neural retina and in the trabecular meshwork. The toxic effect of iron may cause retinal damage and scarring in the trabecular meshwork and a secondary open-angle glaucoma. **B** Distinctive changes in the pigment epithelium are caused by an intraocular iron foreign body. **C** In another case, iron is deposited in the neural retina and in the retinal pigment epithelium. (**A**, Perl's stain; **B**, courtesy of Dr. AJ Brucker; **C**, Perl's stain.)

Labels in figure:
- Non-pigmented ciliary epithelium
- Pigmented ciliary epithelium
- Retinal pigment epithelial changes
- Internal limiting membrane
- Degeneration of inner retinal layers
- Outer nuclear layer
- Retinal pigment epithelium

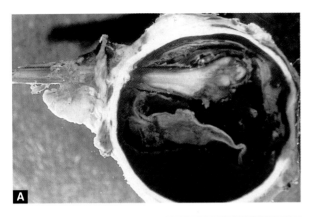

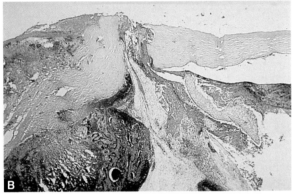

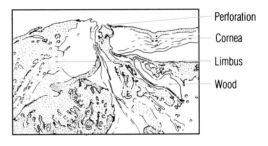

Perforation
Cornea
Limbus
Wood

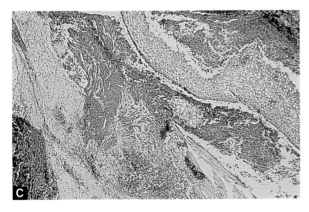

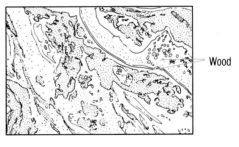

Wood

Fig. 5.38 Intraocular Foreign Body. A The gross specimen shows a large splinter of wood within the eye. **B** Histology shows a perforation through the limbal cornea. The ciliary body, lower left, is filled with blood. Wood (shown under increased magnification in **C**) is present in the anterior chamber and within the wound. (Case courtesy of Dr. WR Green.)

Fig 5.39 INJURIES

Chemical	Burns	Radiation
Acid	Thermal	
Alkali	Electrical	
Tear gas		
Mustard gas		

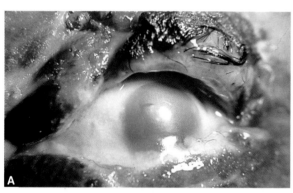

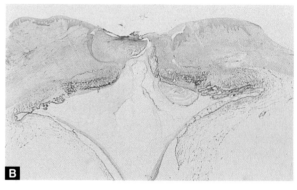

Fig. 5.40   Alkali Burn. A Considerable lye has caused a massive burn to the conjunctiva and cornea in this left eye. The "whiteness" of the eye is a measure of the loss of conjunctiva and is always a bad sign in a lye burn. Ultimately, the cornea became necrotic and perforation occurred. **B** Histologic section of another case shows corneal perforation. Lens remnants, including capsule, are within the corneal wound. Note the thickened cornea and proliferation of corneal epithelium into the stroma. The proliferating epithelium, along with keratocytes and polymorphonuclear leukocytes, secretes collagenase that causes a "melting" of the corneal stroma. The eye is hypotonus, as evidenced by the massive choroidal detachment. (**B,** PAS.)

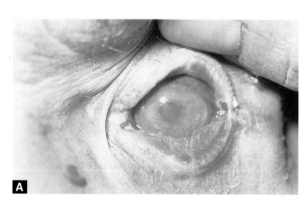

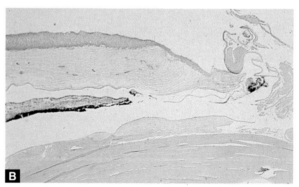

Fig. 5.41   Radiation Injury. A The patient had radiation therapy for sebaceous carcinoma of the eyelid. Note the scarring of the cornea and ciliary injection. **B** Another patient who received radiation therapy for basal cell carcinoma of the eyelid shows corneal perforation. Note the vascularized cornea. Lens remnants and iris are present within the corneal perforation.

Bibliography

Aguilar JP, Green WR: Choroidal rupture. A histopathologic study of 47 cases. Retina 4:269, 1984.

Champion R, Green WE: Intraocular lenses: a histopathologic study of eyes, ocular tissues, and intraocular lenses obtained surgically. Ophthalmology 92:1628, 1985.

Coonan P, et al: The incidence of retinal detachment following extracapsular cataract extraction. A ten-year study. Ophthalmology 92:1096, 1985.

Eagle RC, Yanoff M: Cholesterolosis of the anterior chamber. Albrecht v Graefes Arch klin exp Ophthal 193:121, 1975.

Harris M, et al: Corneal endothelial overgrowth of angle and iris. Evidence of myoblastic differentiation in three cases. Ophthalmology 91:1154, 1984.

Kappelhof JP, et al: An ultrastructural study of Elschnig's pearls in the pseudophakic eye. Am J Ophthalmol 101:58, 1986.

Katz LJ, Cantor LB, Spaeth GL: Complications of surgery in glaucoma. Early and late bacterial endophthalmitis following glaucoma filtration surgery. Ophthalmology 92:959, 1985.

Kozart DM, Eagle RC Jr: Stripping of Descemet's membrane after glaucoma surgery. Ophthalmic Surgery 12:420, 1981.

Kozart DM, Yanoff M, Katowitz JA: Tolerated eyelash embedded in the retina. Arch Ophthalmol 91:235, 1974.

Maumenee AE, Schwartz MF: Acute intraoperative choroidal effusion. Am J Ophthalmol 100:147, 1985.

McDonnell PJ, Patel A, Green WR: Comparison of intracapsular and extracapsular cataract surgery. Histopathologic study of eyes obtained postmortem. Ophthalmology 92:1208, 1985.

Potts AM, Distler JA: Shape factor in the penetration of intraocular foreign bodies. Am J Ophthalmol 100:183, 1985.

Rao GN, Aquavella JV, Goldberg SH, Berk SL: Pseudophakic bullous keratopathy. Relationships to preoperative corneal endothelial status. Ophthalmology 91:1135, 1984.

Sipperly JO, Quigley HA, Gass JDM: Traumatic retinopathy in primates. The explanation of commotio retinae. Arch Ophthalmol 96:2267, 1978.

Tawara A: Transformation and cytotoxicity of iron in siderosis bulbi. Invest Ophthalmol Vis Sci 27:226, 1986.

Tesluk GC, Spaeth GL: The occurrence of primary open-angle glaucoma in the fellow eye of patient with unilateral angle-cleavage glaucoma. Ophthalmology 92:904, 1985.

Yanoff M: In vitro biology of corneal epithelium and endothelium. Trans Am Ophthalmol Soc 73:571, 1975.

Yanoff M, et al: Pathology of human cystoid macular edema. Surv Ophthalmol 28 (Suppl):505, 1984.

LID AND LACRIMAL DRAINAGE SYSTEM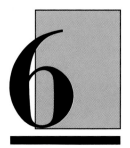

The skin of the eyelids is representative of skin elsewhere in the body. Some conditions, however, either affect the eyelids uniquely or are more common in eyelid structures. The terminology used in dermatopathology will be reviewed where applicable to lid pathology.

Congenital abnormalities may affect the lids alone, or also affect the eyes, or be part of a generalized systemic defect. At the other end of the spectrum, aging changes often involve the eyelids and lead to characteristic and easily defined clinical entities, such as dermatochalasis.

Inflammation commonly involves the eyelids. Although infectious inflammation may occur, allergic conditions are most common. Many of the inflammatory conditions that involve the eyelids have the same histological characteristics as those described previously in Chapters 3 and 4.

Many systemic dermatoses may have lid involvement. The spectrum spans congenital lesions, e.g., ichthyosis congenita; inflammatory conditions, e.g., contact dermatitis; systemic diseases, e.g., collagen diseases; and so forth. The eyelids may be involved alone or may participate in the systemic involvement.

Cysts, pseudoneoplasms, and neoplasms frequently involve the eyelids. The lesions may arise from the surface epithelium, the epidermal appendages, or the dermis. Pigmented tumors of the eyelids are considered in Chapter 17; soft tissue tumors are described mainly in Chapter 14.

The lacrimal drainage system may be involved with congenital abnormalities, inflammation, and tumors. Some of the common entities are discussed below.

FIG. 6.1 NORMAL ANATOMY OF THE LIDS

Skin　　　　　　　　**Subcutaneous tissue**
Epidermis
Dermis

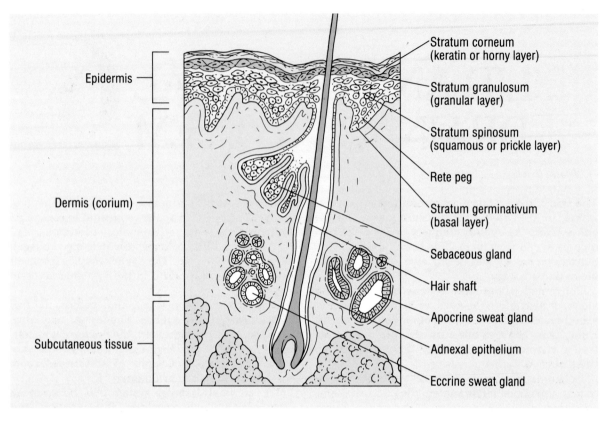

Fig.6.2   Normal Structure of Skin.

Epidermis

Dermis (corium)

Subcutaneous tissue

Stratum corneum (keratin or horny layer)

Stratum granulosum (granular layer)

Stratum spinosum (squamous or prickle layer)

Rete peg

Stratum germinativum (basal layer)

Sebaceous gland

Hair shaft

Apocrine sweat gland

Adnexal epithelium

Eccrine sweat gland

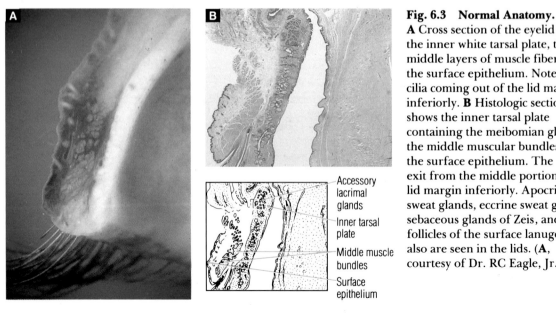

A

B

Accessory lacrimal glands

Inner tarsal plate

Middle muscle bundles

Surface epithelium

Fig. 6.3   Normal Anatomy.
A Cross section of the eyelid shows the inner white tarsal plate, the middle layers of muscle fibers, and the surface epithelium. Note the cilia coming out of the lid margin inferiorly. **B** Histologic section shows the inner tarsal plate containing the meibomian glands, the middle muscular bundles and the surface epithelium. The cilia exit from the middle portion of the lid margin inferiorly. Apocrine sweat glands, eccrine sweat glands, sebaceous glands of Zeis, and hair follicles of the surface lanugo hairs also are seen in the lids. (**A**, courtesy of Dr. RC Eagle, Jr.)

FIG. 6.4 TERMINOLOGY OF EPIDERMIS

Polarity—normal polarity is the orderly arrangement from basal to squamous to granular to keratin layers
Hyperkeratosis—thickening of the keratin layer
Parakeratosis—incomplete keratinization and retention of nuclei in cells of the keratin layer
Acanthosis—increased thickness of the squamous layer
Dyskeratosis—keratinization of individual epithelial cells within the squamous layer
Acantholysis—separation of squamous cells
Bulla—space filled with fluid within or under the epithelium
Atrophy—thinning of the epidermis, diminution of rete pegs, and loss of epidermal appendages
Atypical cell—abnormal cell that, in its extreme, would be cancerous
Leukoplakia—white plaque which has numerous possible causes

FIG. 6.5 CONGENITAL ANOMALIES

Phakomatous choristoma	Epicanthus	Ptosis
Cryptophthalmos	Ectopic caruncle	Ichthyosis congenita
Microblepharon	Lid margin anomalies	Xeroderma pigmentosum
Coloboma	Eyelash anomalies	

FIG. 6.6 AGING

Atrophy
Dermatochalasis
Herniation of the orbital fat

FIG. 6.7 INFLAMMATION

Hordeolum
External (stye)
Internal
Chalazion
Acne rosacea

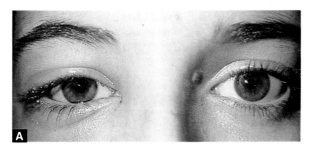

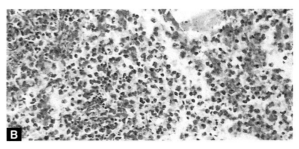

Fig. 6.8   Hordeolum. A The patient complained of swelling, redness, and pain of the left lower lid of a few days' duration. The inflammation is located mainly in the outer layers of the lid and is called an external hordeolum. Similar inflammation in the inner layers is called an internal hordeolum.
B Histologic section of another case shows a purulent exudate consisting of polymorphonuclear leukocytes and cellular debris.

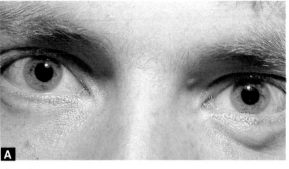

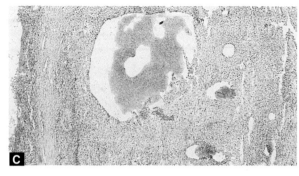

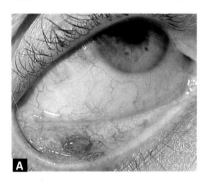

Fig. 6.9   Chalazion. A A hard, painless lump was present within the left lower lid for at least a few weeks. B Histologic section shows a clear, circular area surrounded by epithelioid cells and multinucleated giant cells. In processing the tissue, fat is dissolved out, and the area where fat had been appears clear.
C Fresh frozen tissue that has not been processed through solvents stains positively for fat in the circular areas. (C, oil red-O.)

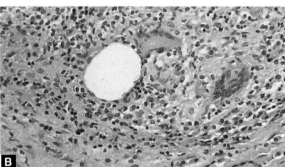

Fig. 6.10   Granuloma Pyogenicum. A The patient who had had a hard, painless lump in the right lower lid for over a month came in complaining of the red, fleshy area inside the lid.
B Histologic section shows a vascularized tissue (granulation tissue) that consists of inflammatory cells, fibroblasts, and the endothelial cells of budding capillaries.

Polymorpho-
nuclear
leukocytes

Endothelial
cells

Capillaries

Plasma cell

Fibroblast

FIG. 6.11 VIRAL DISEASES

Molluscum contagiosum
Verruca vulgaris (wart)
Vesicular lesions
Variola (smallpox)
Varicella (chicken pox)
Herpes zoster (shingles)
Herpes simplex (cold sore)
Trachoma
*Lymphogranuloma
venereum*

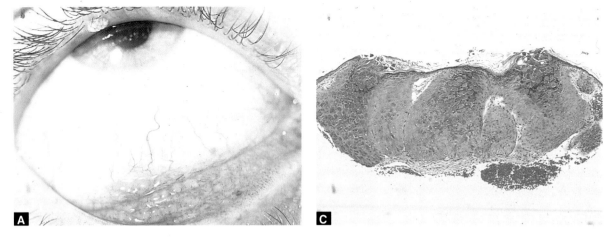

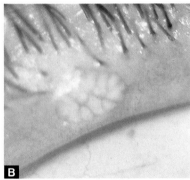

Fig. 6.12 *Molluscum contagiosum.* **A** A follicular conjunctivitis is present in the inferior, bulbar conjunctiva. Note the small lesion on the margin of the superior eyelid that is responsible for the follicular conjunctivitis. **B** Increased magnification demonstrates an umbilicated lesion that contains whitish packets of material. **C** Histologic section shows that the epithelium is thickened by intracytoplasmic *Molluscum* bodies that are small and eosinophilic in the deep layers but become enormous and basophilic near the surface. After breaking through the surface epithelium, the *Molluscum* bodies may be shed into the tear film where they cause a secondary, irritative, follicular conjunctivitis. (**A** and **B**; courtesy Dr. WC Frayer.)

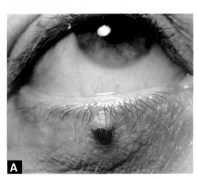

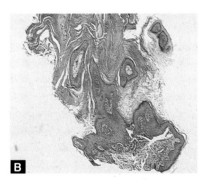

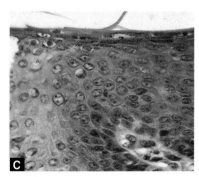

Fig. 6.13 *Verruca vulgaris.* **A** Clinical appearance of lesion. **B** Histologic section shows marked hyperkeratosis. Note that the rete ridges are elongated and bent inward, a rather typical finding. **C** Another area shows deeply basophilic inclusion bodies and vacuolated cells. Inclusion bodies are often found near the vacuolated cells.

FIG. 6.14 BACTERIAL DISEASES

Impetigo
Staphylococcus
Parinaud's oculoglandular
   syndrome (see Chapter 7)
(Fungal and parasitic diseases
   see Chapter 4)

FIG. 6.15 MANIFESTATIONS OF SYSTEMIC PROBLEMS

Ichthyosis congenita
Xeroderma pigmentosum
Pemphigus
Erythema multiforme
Ehlers–Danlos syndrome
Cutis laxa
Pseudoxanthoma elasticum
Toxic epidermal necrolysis
Contact dermatitis
Collagen diseases

Xanthelasma
Juvenile xanthogranuloma (see
   Chapter 9)
Amyloidosis (see Chapter 7)
Calcinosis cutis
Lipoid proteinosis
Hemochromatosis
Relapsing febrile nodular
   nonsuppurative panniculitis

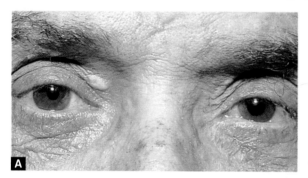

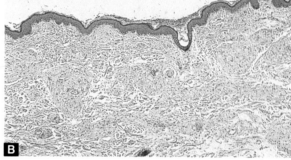

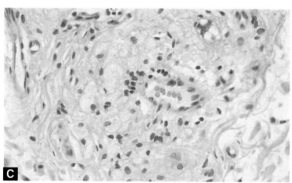

Fig. 6.16   Xanthelasma. A The inner aspect of each upper lid (greater on the right upper lid) is thickened by a fatty deposit in the dermis.
B Histologic section of xanthelasma shows thickening of the dermis by clusters of lipid-filled macrophages.
C The lipid-filled macrophages tend to cluster around blood vessels. The material within the macrophages stains positively for fat.

FIG. 6.17 BENIGN CYSTIC LESIONS

Epidermoid and dermoid cysts
   (see Chapter 14)
Epithelial inclusion cyst
Sebaceous cyst

Comedo (blackhead)
Ductal cysts

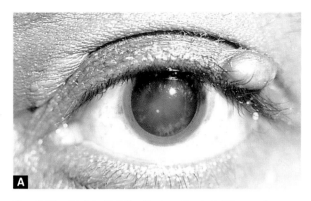

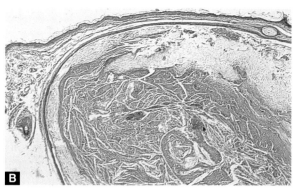

Fig. 6.18 Epithelial Inclusion Cyst. A The patient has a large, epithelial inclusion cyst of the outer third of the left upper lid. Note the xanthelasma at the inner corner of the left upper lid. **B** The cyst is lined by stratified squamous epithelium that desquamates keratin into its lumen.

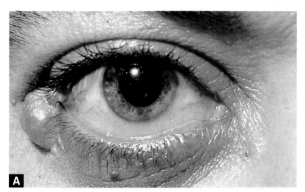

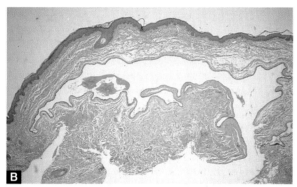

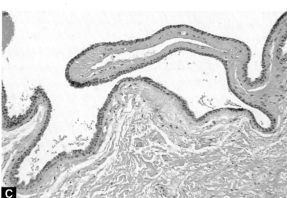

Fig. 6.19 Ductal Cyst. A Ductal cyst noted near outer margin of the right lower lid. **B** The multiloculated cyst is lined by a double-layered epithelium, shown with increased magnification in **C**.

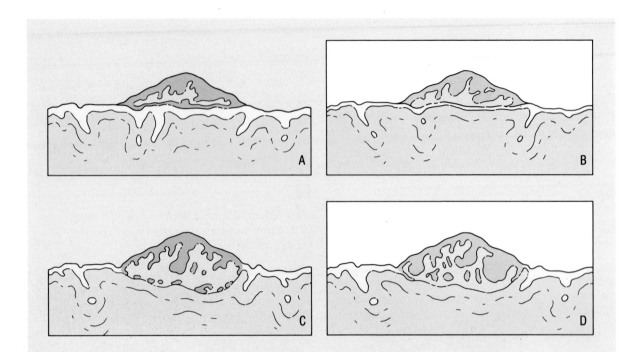

Fig. 6.20 Differences Between Benign and Malignant Skin Lesions. A An elevated lesion sitting as a 'button' on the skin surface. This is characteristic of benign papillomatous lesions. Such lesions, when red, show acanthosis, such as in actinic keratosis. **B** Lesions structurally similar to **A** but that appear blue under low magnification are caused by proliferation of basal cells, as in seborrheic keratosis. **C** An elevated lesion that invades the underlying skin is characteristic of a malignancy. Invasive lesions that appear red under low magnification are caused by a proliferation of the squamous layer (acanthosis), as in squamous cell carcinoma. **D** A lesion structurally similar to **C** but that appears blue under low magnification represents proliferation of basal cells, as seen in basal cell carcinoma.

FIG. 6.21 BENIGN TUMORS OF SURFACE EPITHELIUM

Papilloma
Nevus verrucosis (Jadassohn)
Actinic keratosis
Verruca vulgaris
Seborrheic keratosis
Acanthosis nigricans
Squamous papilloma

Inverted follicular keratosis
Pseudoepitheliomatous
   hyperplasia
Keratoacanthoma
Others
Benign keratosis

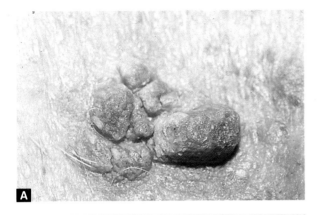

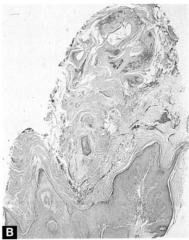

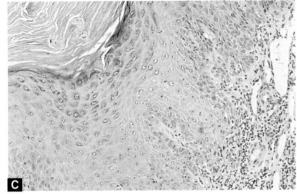

Fig. 6.22 Actinic Keratosis. A The clinical appearance of a lesion involving the left upper lid. **B** Histologic section shows a papillomatous lesion that is above the skin surface, appears red in color, and has marked hyperkeratosis and acanthosis. **C** Although the squamous layer of the skin is increased in thickness (acanthosis) and the basal layer shows atypical cells, the normal polarity of the epidermis is preserved.

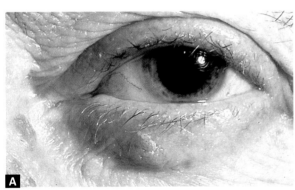

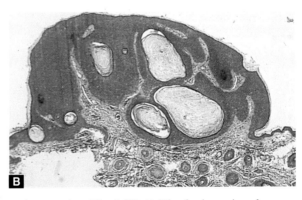

Fig. 6.23 Seborrheic Keratosis. A A "greasy" elevated lesion is present in the middle, nasal portion of the left lower lid. Biopsy showed this to be a seborrheic keratosis. The smaller lesion just inferior and nasal to the seborrheic keratosis proved to be a syringoma (see Fig. 6.38). **B** Histologic section shows a papillomatous lesion that lies above the skin surface and is blue in color. The lesion contains proliferated basaloid cells and keratin-filled cysts.

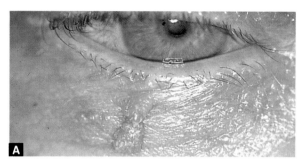

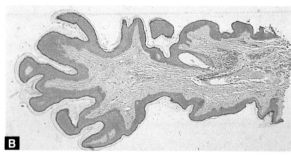

Fig. 6.24 Squamous Papilloma. A A skin tag is noted in the middle portion of the lower lid. **B** Histologic section shows a narrow-based papilloma that contains many finger-like processes called fronds. The fronds are covered by an acanthotic, hyperkeratotic epithelium and contain a fibrovascular core.

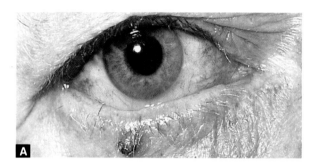

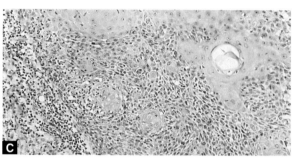

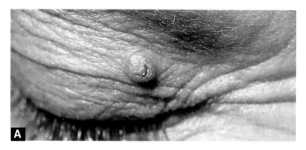

Fig. 6.25 Inverted Follicular Keratosis. A Clinical appearance of lesion in the middle of the right lower lid. **B** Histologic section shows a papillomatous lesion above the skin surface composed mainly of acanthotic epithelium. **C** Increased magnification shows separation or acantholysis of individual squamous cells that surround the characteristic squamous eddies.

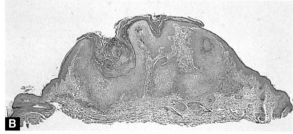

Fig. 6.26 Keratoacanthoma. A This patient had a 6-week history of a rapidly enlarging lesion. Note the umbilicated central area. **B** Histologic section shows that the lesion is above the surface epithelium, has a cup-shaped configuration, and a central keratin core. The base of the acanthotic epithelium is blunted (rather than invasive) at the junction of the dermis.

FIG. 6.28 CANCEROUS TUMORS OF SURFACE EPITHELIUM

Basal cell carcinoma
Squamous cell carcinoma (rare)
Intraepidermal
Invasive

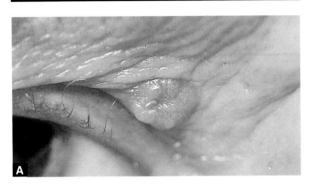

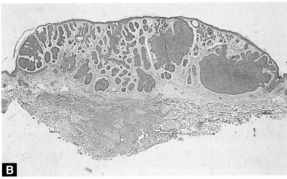

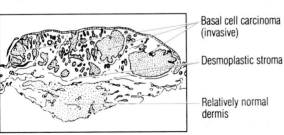

Basal cell carcinoma (invasive)

Desmoplastic stroma

Relatively normal dermis

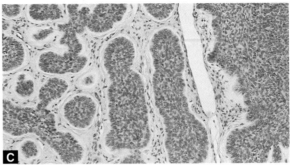

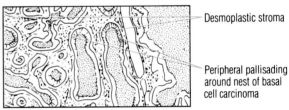

Desmoplastic stroma

Peripheral pallisading around nest of basal cell carcinoma

Fig. 6.29   Basal Cell Carcinoma. A A firm, indurated, painless lesion had been present for about 8 months. **B** Excisional biopsy shows epithelial proliferation arising from the basal layer of the epidermis. The proliferated cells appear blue and are present in nests of different sizes. Note the sharp demarcation of the pale, pink area of stroma supporting the neoplastic cells from the underlying (normal) dark pink dermis. This stromal change, called desmoplasia, is characteristic of neoplastic lesions. Compare with the benign lesions in Figs. 6.23–6.25, where the dermis does not show such a change. **C** The nests are composed of atypical basal cells and show peripheral palisading. Mitotic figures are present. Again, note the pseudosarcomatous change (desmoplasia) of the surrounding supporting stroma which is light pink and contains proliferating fibroblasts. (**A** courtesy of Dr. HG Scheie.)

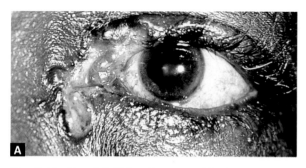

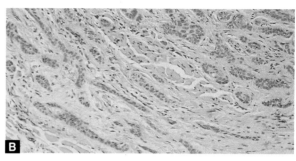

Fig. 6.30 Basal Cell Carcinoma. A The inner aspect of the eyelids are ulcerated by the infiltrating tumor. **B** Histologic section shows the morphea-like or fibrosing type, where the basal cells grow in thin strands or cords, often only one cell layer thick, closely resembling metastatic scirrhous carcinoma of the breast ("indian file" pattern). This uncommon type of basal cell carcinoma has a much worse prognosis than the more common type.

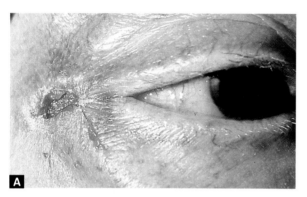

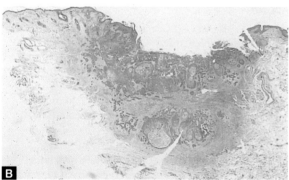

Fig. 6.31 Squamous Cell Carcinoma. A The patient has an ulcerating lesion of the lateral aspect of the eyelids that had increased in size over many months. **B** Histologic section of the excisional biopsy shows epithelial cells, with an overall pink color, which infiltrate the dermis deeply. The overlying region is ulcerated. **C** Increased magnification shows the squamous neoplastic cells making keratin (horn cyst) in an abnormal location (dyskeratosis). Numerous mitotic figures are present. Note the pseudosarcomatous (dysplastic) change in the surrounding stroma.

FIG. 6.32 TUMORS OF SEBACEOUS GLANDS

Congenital sebaceous gland hyperplasia	Sebaceous adenoma
Acquired sebaceous gland hyperplasia	Sebaceous gland carcinoma
Adenoma sebaceum of Pringle (angiofibroma of face)	

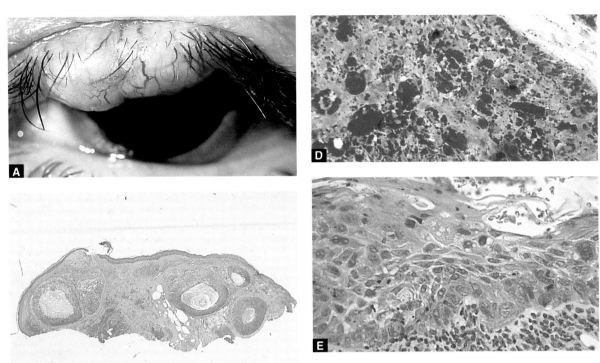

Fig. 6.33 Sebaceous Cell Carcinoma. A Clinical appearance of lesion that simulates a large chalazion. Note the characteristic loss of hair over the lesion. **B** Histologic section shows large tumor nodules, most of which exhibit central necrosis, in the dermis. **C** Increased magnification shows that numerous cells resemble sebaceous gland cells. A number of mitotic figures are present. **D** Many of the cells stain positively for fat. Any recurrent or suspicious chalazion should be biopsied. **E** In another case, large tumor cells are scattered throughout the epithelium, resembling Paget's disease and called pagetoid change. The cancerous invasion of the epithelium can cause a chronic, nongranulomatous, blepharoconjunctivitis (masquerade syndrome). (**D**, oil red-O).

FIG. 6.34 TUMORS OF HAIR FOLLICLES

Trichoepithelioma (Brooke's tumor)
Trichofolliculoma
Trichilemmoma

Pilomatrixoma (calcifying epithelioma of Malherbe)
Merkel cell tumor
Adnexal carcinoma

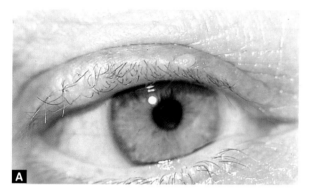

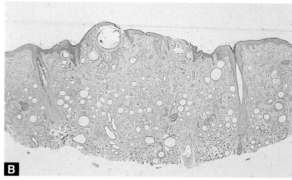

Fig. 6.35 Trichoepithelioma. A Clinical appearance of a lesion in the middle of the right upper lid near the margin. **B** Histologic section shows the tumor diffusely present throughout the dermis. The tumor is composed of multiple, squamous cell horn cysts that represent immature hair structures.

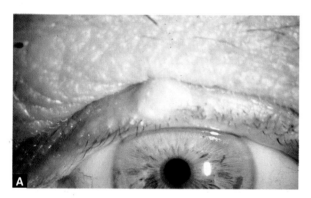

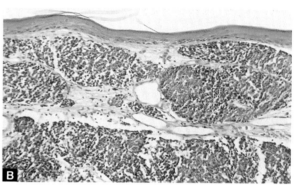

Fig. 6.36 Merkel Cell Tumor. A Clinical appearance of a lesion in the middle portion of the upper lid. **B** Histologic section shows nests of dark, poorly differentiated cells in the dermis. Mitotic figures also are seen. The tumor appears to arise from cells, commonly associated with hair follicles that form complexes with terminal neurites, acting as a specific, sensory, epithelial, nerve cell receptor. (Case presented in 1985 to the Eastern Ophthalmic Pathology Society by Dr. DA Morris.)

FIG. 6.37 TUMORS OF SWEAT GLANDS

Syringoma
Syringocystadenoma papilleferum
Eccrine spiradenoma
Eccrine mixed tumor
Cylindroma (Turban tumor)
Eccrine poroma
Sweat gland carcinoma

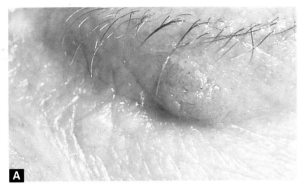

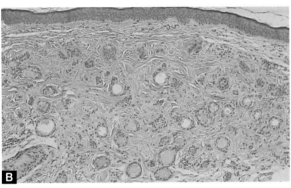

Fig. 6.38 Syringoma. A Clinical appearance of lesions just below and nasal to seborrheic keratosis of left lower lid (see same patient illustrated in Fig. 6.23). **B** Histologic section shows that the dermis contains proliferated eccrine sweat structures that form epithelial strands and cystic spaces. **C** Increased magnification demonstrates epithelial strands and cystic spaces that are lined by a double-layered epithelium.

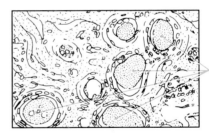

Surface epithelium

Tumor "ducts" and epithelial Strands

Cystic spaces lined by double-layered epithelium

FIG. 6.39 OTHER EYELID TUMORS	FIG. 6.40 LACRIMAL DRAINAGE SYSTEM	
Metastatic tumors	**Congenital abnormalities**	**Tumors**
Pigmented tumors (see Chapter 17)	Atresia of nasolacrimal duct	Epithelial
Mesenchymal tumors (see Chapter 14)	Atresia of punctum	Papillomas: squamous, transitional, or adenoma
	Fistula of lacrimal sac	Carcinoma: squamous, transitional, or adenoma
	Inflammation	Melanotic (see Chapter 17)
		Mesenchymal (see Chapter 14)

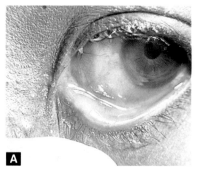

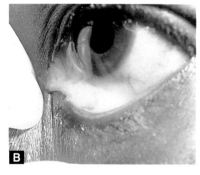

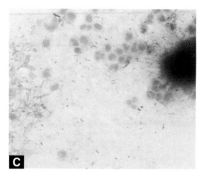

Fig. 6.41   Dacryocystitis. A and **B** The patient had a history of tearing and a lump in the region of the lacrimal sac. Pressure over the lacrimal sac shows increasing amounts of pus coming through the punctum. **C** Another patient had an acute canaliculitis. Smear of the lacrimal cast obtained at biopsy shows large colonies of delicate, branching, intertwined filaments characteristic of *Streptothrix* (*Actinomyces*).

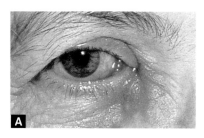

Fig. 6.42   Squamous Cell Carcinoma of the Lacrimal Sac. A Clinical appearance of tumor in region of right lacrimal sac. **B** Strands and cords of cells are infiltrating the tissues surrounding the lacrimal sac. **C** Increased magnification shows the cells to be undifferentiated, malignant, squamous cells. (Case presented by Dr. AG Spalding at 1982 Verhoeff Society Meeting.)

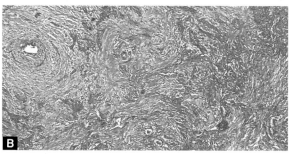

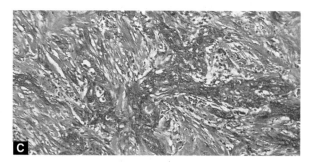

Bibliography

Arnold AC, Bullock JD, Foos RY: Metastatic eyelid carcinoma. Ophthalmology 92:114, 1985.

Boniuk M, Zimmerman LE: Eyelid tumors with reference to lesions confused with squamous cell carcinoma. III. Keratoacanthoma. Arch Ophthalmol 77:29, 1967.

Doxanas MT, Green WR: Sebaceous gland carcinoma. Review of 40 cases. Arch Ophthalmol 102:245, 1984.

Friedman AH, Henkind P: Granuloma pyogenicum of the palpebral conjunctiva. Am J Ophthalmol 71:868, 1971.

Glatt HJ, et al: Malignant syringoma of the eyelid. Ophthalmology 91:987, 1984.

Hidyat A, Font RL: Trichilemmoma of eyelid and eyebrow. A clinicopathologic study of 31 cases. Arch Ophthalmol 98:844, 1980.

Middelkamp JN, Munger BL: Ultrastructure and histogenesis of Molluscum contagiosum. J Pediatr 64:888, 1964.

Perlman GS, Hornblass A: Basal cell carcinoma of the eyelids: a review of patients treated by surgical excision. Ophthal Surg 7:23, 1976.

Rao NA, et al: Sebaceous carcinomas of the ocular adnexa: a clinicopathologic study of 104 cases, with five-year follow-up data. Hum Pathol 13:113, 1982.

Ryan SJ, Font RL: Primary epithelial neoplasms of the lacrimal sac. Am J Ophthalmol 76:73, 1973.

Searle SS, et al: Malignant Merkel cell neoplasm of the eyelid. Arch Ophthalmol 102:907, 1984.

Spielvogel RL, Austin C, Ackerman AB: Inverted follicular keratosis is not a specific keratosis but a verruca vulgaris (or seborrheic keratosis) with squamous eddies. Am J Dermatopathol 5:427, 1983.

CONJUNCTIVA 7

The conjunctiva is a mucous membrane, similar to mucous membranes elsewhere in the body. Congenital anomalies and vascular disorders may involve the conjunctiva, but they are unusual and relatively unimportant from a pathological point of view. Inflammation of the conjunctiva is one of the most common entities that bring patients to the ophthalmologist. The basic principles of the pathology of inflammation have been covered in Chapters 3 and 4. One group of organisms, the chlamydias, especially the one that causes trachoma, is responsible for a significant proportion of human blindness and is illustrated here. Injuries are discussed in Chapter 5.

Manifestations of systemic diseases may be seen in the conjunctiva. For example, metabolic products may be deposited, as in ochronosis. Vitamin A deficiency may cause xerosis or a Bitot's spot. Numerous skin diseases also may involve the conjunctiva.

Degenerations, especially pinguecula and pterygium, are extremely common in the conjunctiva. Cysts, either congenital or acquired, are also commonly seen.

The epithelium of the conjunctiva may undergo both benign and malignant proliferations. Stromal neoplasms may also occur, but these are similar to those that occur in the orbit and are considered in Chapter 14. Pigmented lesions of the conjunctiva are discussed with other pigmented lesions in and about the eye in Chapter 17.

FIG. 7.1 CONGENITAL ANOMALIES

Cryptophthalmos (ablepharon)
Epitarsus
Hereditary hemorrhagic telangiectasia (Rendu–Osler–Weber syndrome)
Congenital conjunctival lymphedema (Nonne–Milroy–Meige disease)
Dermoids, epidermoids, dermolipomas

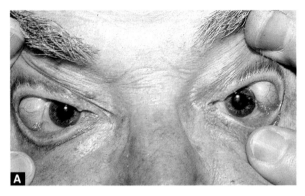

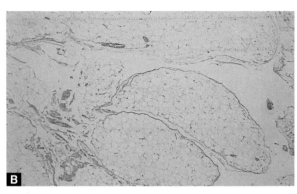

Fig. 7.2 Dermolipoma. A The patient shows the typical clinical appearance of bilateral, temporal dermolipomas. **B** The histologic specimen shows that the dermolipoma is composed almost completely of fatty tissue. Rarely, dermolipomas may also show structures, such as epidermal appendages and fibrous tissue.

FIG. 7.3 INFLAMMATION: CELLS OF CONJUNCTIVITIS

Predominant cells	Type of conjunctivitis
Polymorphonuclear leukocyte	Bacterial
Eosinophils and basophils	Allergic
Mononuclear cells (mainly lymphocytes)	Viral
Multinucleated giant cells	Herpes, rubella, tuberculosis

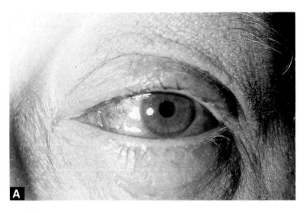

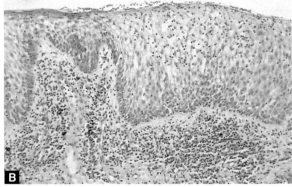

Fig. 7.4 Acute Conjunctivitis. A Clinical appearance of a mucopurulent conjunctivitis of the left eye. **B** The major inflammatory cell of acute, bacterial conjunctivitis is the polymorphonuclear leukocyte, which here infiltrates the swollen, edematous epithelium and the substantia propria.

FIG. 7.5 INFLAMMATION: INFLAMMATORY MEMBRANES

True membrane
When removed, epithelium is also removed, leaving a bleeding surface
Seen in epidemic keratoconjunctivitis (EKC), *Corynebacterium diphtheriae,* Stevens–Johnson syndrome, *Pneumococcus,* and *Staphylococcus aureus*

Pseudomembrane
When removed, epithelium is not disturbed
Seen in EKC, *Corynebacterium diphtheriae,* Stevens–Johnson syndrome, *Streptococcus hemolyticus,* pharyngoconjunctival fever, vernal conjunctivitis, ligneous conjunctivitis, and alkali burns

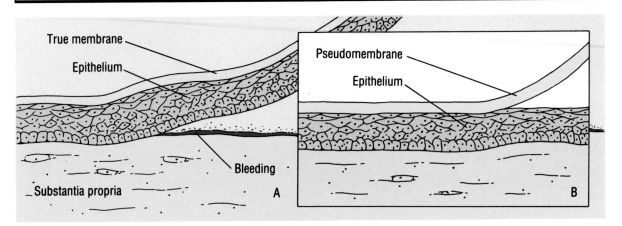

Fig. 7.6   Inflammatory Membranes. A In a true membrane, when the membrane is stripped off, the epithelium is also removed and a bleeding surface is left. **B** In a pseudomembrane, when the membrane is stripped off, it comes off the epithelium, leaving the epithelium intact and no bleeding takes place.

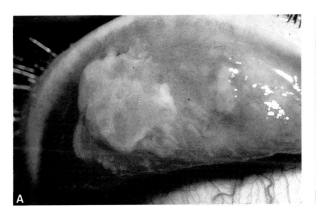

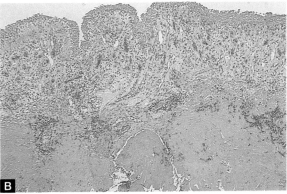

Fig. 7.7   Ligneous Conjunctivitis. A A thick membrane covers the upper palpebral conjunctiva. **B** Biopsy shows a thick, amorphous material contiguous with an inflammatory membrane composed mostly of mononuclear inflammatory cells (mainly plasma cells and some lymphocytes). (Case presented by Dr. J.S. McGavic at the Verhoeff Society, 1986.)

FIG. 7.8 INFLAMMATION: CHRONIC CONJUNCTIVITIS

Hyperplastic epithelium
Follicular hypertrophy
Papillary hypertrophy
Granuloma pyogenicum
Granulomatous inflammation

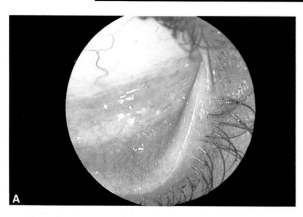

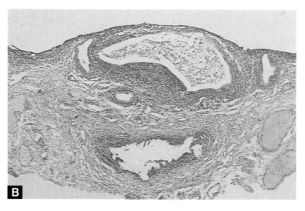

Fig. 7.9   Chronic Conjunctivitis. A The conjunctiva is thickened and contains tiny yellow cysts.
B Histologic section of the conjunctiva demonstrates the cyst lined by an epithelium which resembles ductal epithelium and contains a pink, granular material. A chronic, nongranulomatous inflammation of lymphocytes and plasma cells surrounds the cyst, along with a proliferation of the epithelium of the palpebral conjunctiva, forming structures which resemble glands and are called pseudoglands (Henle).

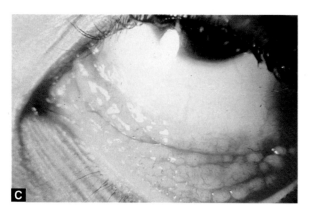

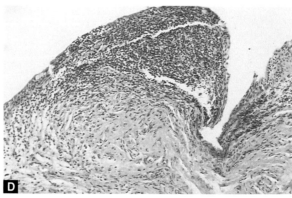

Fig. 7.10   Follicular Conjunctivitis. A The surfaces of the follicles are pale, whereas their bases are red.
B Histologic section of the conjunctiva shows a lymphoid follicle in the substantia propria.

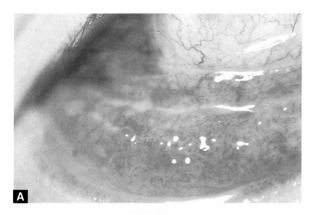

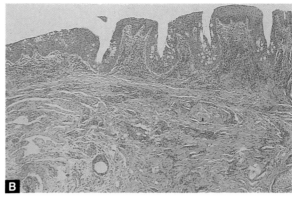

Fig. 7.11 Papillary Conjunctivitis. A The surfaces of the papillae are red because of numerous tiny vessels, whereas their bases are pale in color. **B** Histologic section of the conjunctiva demonstrates an inflammatory infiltrate in the substantia propria and numerous small vessels coursing through the papillae. The inflammatory cells are lymphocytes and plasma cells.

FIG. 7.12 INFLAMMATION: SCARRING

Ocular pemphigoid
Secondary, e.g., to Stevens–Johnson syndrome or alkali burns

FIG. 7.13 INFLAMMATION: SPECIFIC INFLAMMATION

Bacterial
Viral
Chlamydias
Trachoma
Inclusion conjunctivitis
Lymphogranuloma venereum
Ornithosis (psittacosis)
Fungal
Parasitic
Rickettsial
Parinaud's oculoglandular syndrome
Chemical injuries
Vernal keratoconjunctivitis

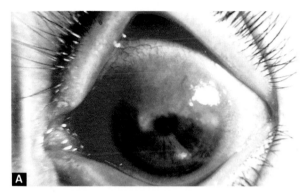

Fig. 7.14 Trachoma. A The patient has a trachomatous pannus growing over the superior conjunctiva. With healing, the follicles disappear from the peripheral cornea, leaving areas filled with a thickened, transparent epithelium called Herbert's pits. The palpebral conjunctiva scars by the formation of a white, linear, horizontal line or scar near the upper border of the tarsus called von Arlt's line. **B** A conjunctival smear from another case of trachoma shows a large, cytoplasmic, basophilic, initial body. Small, cytoplasmic, elementary bodies are seen in some of the other cells. **C** Small, cytoplasmic, elementary bodies are seen in numerous cells. (**A**, courtesy of Dr. AP Ferry.)

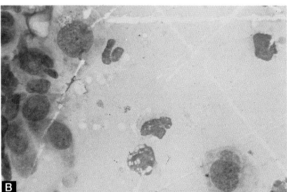

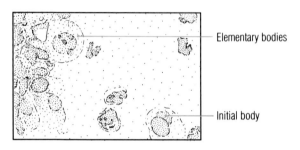

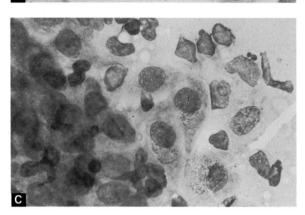

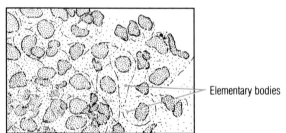

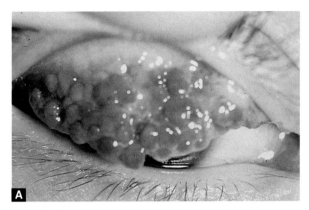

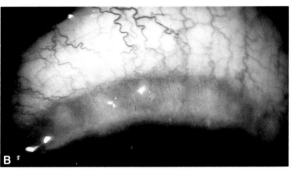

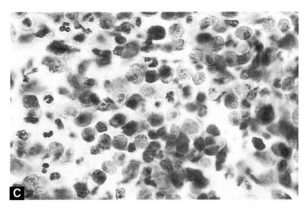

Fig. 7.15 Vernal Catarrh. A Clinical appearance of the papillary reaction of the palpebral conjunctiva. **B** Clinical appearance of the less commonly seen limbal reaction. **C** Histologic examination of a conjunctival smear shows the presence of many eosinophils. (**B** and **C**, courtesy of Dr. IM Raber.)

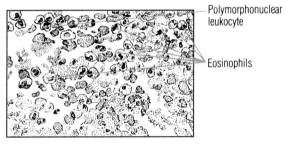

Polymorphonuclear leukocyte

Eosinophils

FIG. 7.16 MANIFESTATIONS OF SYSTEMIC DISEASE: DEPOSITION OF METABOLIC PRODUCTS

Cystinosis	Mucopolysaccharidoses	Porphyria
Ochronosis	Lipoidoses	Jaundice
Hypercalcemia	Dysproteinemias	Degos' disease
Addison's disease		

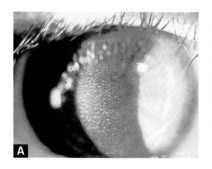
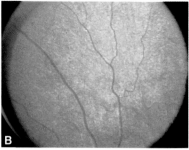
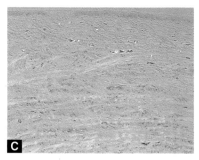

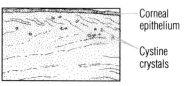

Corneal
epithelium

Cystine
crystals

Fig. 7.17   Cystinosis. A Clinical appearance of cystine crystals in the cornea. **B** Deposition of cystine in the retinal pigment epithelium and choroid gives the fundus a crystalloid appearance. **C** Polarization of an unstained histologic section of cornea shows the birefringent, cystine crystals. (**A** and **B**, courtesy of Dr. DB Schaffer.)

FIG. 7.18 MANIFESTATIONS OF SYSTEMIC DISEASE: DEPOSITION OF DRUG DERIVATIVES

Argyrosis	Atabrine	Mercury
Chlorpromazine	Epinephrine	Arsenicals

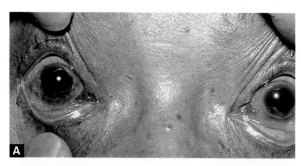

Fig. 7.19   Argyrosis. A Patient had taken silver-containing drops for many years. Note the slate-gray appearance of conjunctiva. **B** The cornea shows a diffuse granular appearance. **C** The granular, corneal appearance is caused by silver deposition in Descemet's membrane. **D** Histologic section shows silver deposited in the epithelium and in the mucosal basement membrane of the lacrimal sac. (**D**, modified from Yanoff M and Scheie HG: Arch Ophthalmol 72:57, 1964.)

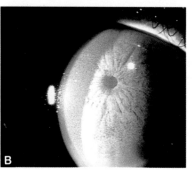
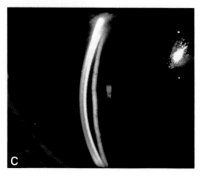
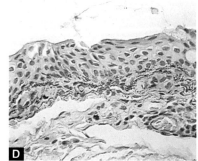

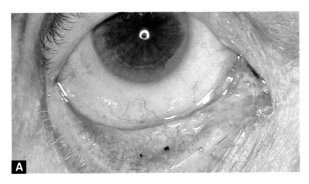

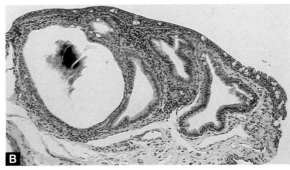

Fig. 7.20 Epinephrine Deposition. A Black spots in palpebral conjunctiva represent the deposition of epinephrine after long-term use in the treatment of glaucoma. **B** Histologic section shows that the material within a cyst in the epithelium has properties similar to melanin. The stain here is a Fontana stain that characteristically stains silver/dark brown.

FIG. 7.21 DEGENERATIONS

Xerosis	Pinguecula	Amyloidosis
Pterygium (see Chapter 8)	Lipid deposits	

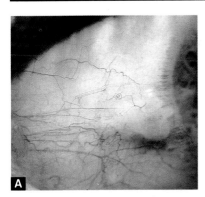

Fig. 7.22 Pinguecula. A A pinguecula characteristically involves the limbal conjunctiva, most frequently nasally, and appears as a white-yellowish mound of tissue. **B** Histologic section shows basophilic degeneration of the conjunctival substantia propria. **C** Another case shows even more marked basophilic degeneration that stains heavily black when a stain for elastic tissue is used. (**C**, Verhoeff's elastica.)

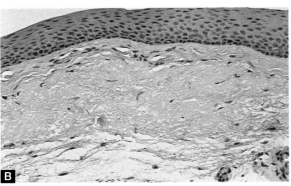

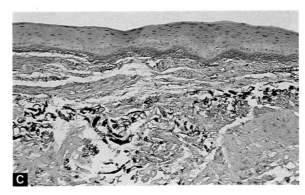

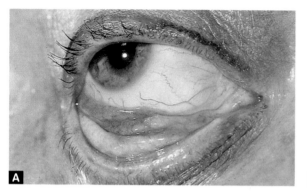

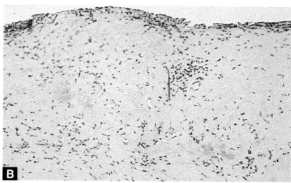

Fig. 7.23 Amyloidosis. A The patient has a smooth, fish-flesh, redundant mass in the inferior conjunctiva of both eyes, present for many years. The underlying cause was unknown, and the patient had no systemic involvement. Clinically, this could be lymphoid hyperplasia, lymphoma, leukemia, or amyloidosis. The lesion was biopsied. **B** Histologic section shows an amorphous, pale, hyaline deposit in the substantia propria of the conjunctiva that stains positively with the Congo red stain. The scant inflammatory cellular infiltrate consists mainly of lymphocytes, plasma cells, and mast cells. (**B**, Congo red; case reported in Glass R, et al: Ann Ophthalmol 3:823, 1971.)

FIG. 7.24 TUMORS	
Epithelial cysts	**Hamartomas**
Epidermoid	Lymphangioma
Dermoid	Hemangioma
Dermolipoma	Phacomatoses (see Chapter 2)
Ductal	
Inflammatory	

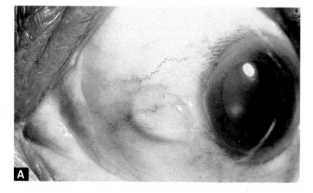

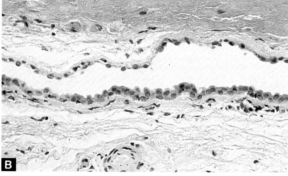

Fig. 7.25 Conjunctival Cyst. A A clear cyst is present just nasal to the limbus. **B** Histologic section of another clear, conjunctival cyst shows that it is lined by a double layer of epithelium, suggesting a ductal origin.

FIG. 7.26 TUMORS (continued)

Pseudocancerous epithelial lesions
Hereditary benign intraepithelial dyskeratosis
Pseudoepitheliomatous hyperplasia
Papilloma
Eosinophilic cystadenoma (oncocytoma)

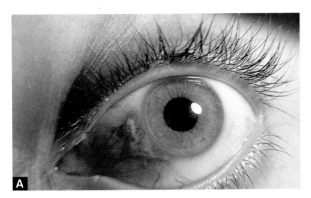

Fig. 7.27   Hereditary Benign Intraepithelial Dyskeratosis (HBID). A The patient has an obvious nasal vascularized, pearly lesion in her left eye. The right eye was quite similar. The patient's mother also had similar lesions. **B** Histologic section shows an acanthotic epithelium that contains dyskeratotic cells. (**B**, case reported in Yanoff M: Arch Ophthalmol 79:291, 1968.)

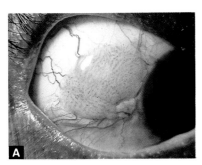

Fig. 7.28   Papilloma. A A large, sessile papilloma of the limbal conjunctiva is present. **B** Histologic section shows a papillary lesion composed of acanthotic epithelium and many blood vessels going into the individual fronds. The base of the lesion is quite broad. **C** Increased magnification shows the blood vessels and the acanthotic epithelium. Although the epithelium is thickened, the polarity from basal cell to surface cell is normal and shows an appropriate transition. (**A**, courtesy of Dr. DM Kozart.)

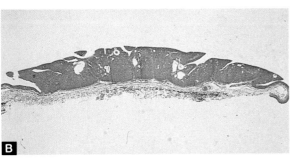

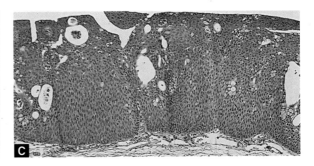

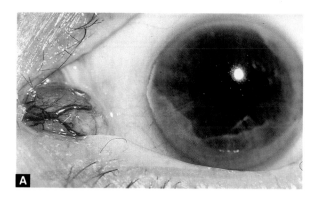

Fig. 7.29 Eosinophilic Cystadenoma (Oncocytoma, Oxyphilic Cell Adenoma). A A fleshy, vascularized lesion is present at the caruncle. **B** Histologic section shows proliferating epithelium around a cystic cavity. **C** Increased magnification shows large, eosinophilic cells which resemble apocrine cells and are forming gland-like spaces. (**A**, courtesy of Dr. HG Scheie.)

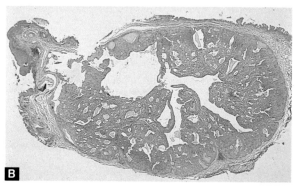

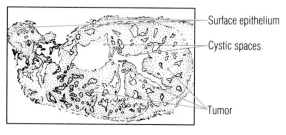

Surface epithelium

Cystic spaces

Tumor

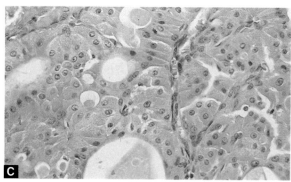

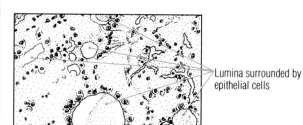

Lumina surrounded by epithelial cells

FIG. 7.30 TUMORS (continued)

Precancerous epithelial lesions
Xeroderma pigmentosum
Actinic keratosis
Dysplasia

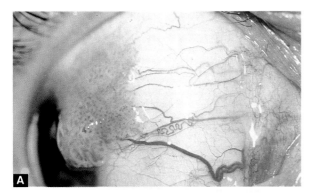

Fig. 7.31 Papilloma With Dysplasia. A Clinical appearance of typical, limbal, sessile, conjunctival papilloma. **B** Histologic section shows a sudden and abrupt transition from the normal conjunctival epithelium to a markedly thickened epithelium. The lesion is broad based and shows numerous blood vessels penetrating into the thickened epithelium. **C** Increased magnification shows a tissue with normal polarity but which contains atypical cells and individual cells making keratin (dyskeratosis). Because the polarity is normal, a diagnosis of dysplasia was made.

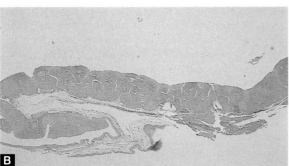

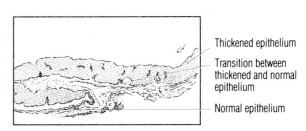

Thickened epithelium

Transition between thickened and normal epithelium

Normal epithelium

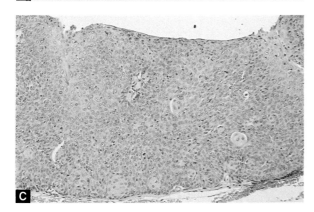

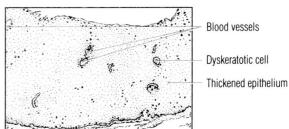

Blood vessels

Dyskeratotic cell

Thickened epithelium

FIG. 7.32 TUMORS (continued)

Cancerous epithelial lesions
Carcinoma *in situ*
Squamous cell carcinoma, invasive
Basal cell carcinoma (rare)
Carcinoma derived from mucus-secreting cells (rare)

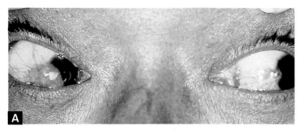

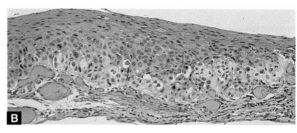

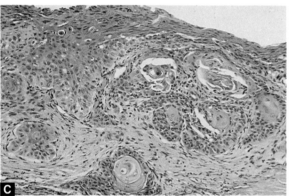

Fig. 7.33 Squamous Cell Carcinoma. A The patient had a vascularized, elevated, pearly lesion at the temporal limbus in the right eye. In addition, he had a pterygium nasally in the left eye. Excisional biopsy of the lesion in the right eye was diagnosed as carcinoma *in situ*. **B** Histologic section of another case shows full thickness atypia, and loss of polarity. A diagnosis of carcinoma *in situ* would be made here. **C** Other regions of this case show malignant epithelial cells in the substantia propria of the conjunctiva, forming keratin pearls in some areas representing invasive squamous cell carcinoma.

FIG. 7.34 TUMORS (continued)

Pigmented tumors (see Chapter 17)
Stromal neoplasms (see Chapter 14)
Angiomatous
Inflammatory pseudotumors, lymphomas,
    leukemias
Juvenile xanthogranuloma (JXG)
Neural, fibrous, and muscle tumors
Metastatic

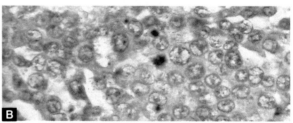

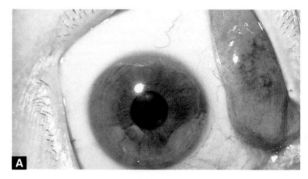

Fig. 7.35 Leukemia. A The patient has a smooth, "fish-flesh" lesion that had appeared a few weeks previously. A diagnosis of acute leukemia had recently been made. **B** Histologic section shows sheets of immature, blastic leukemic cells, many of which are engaged in mitotic activity.

Bibliography

Borodic GE, et al: Immunoglobulin deposition in localized conjunctival amyloidosis. Am J Ophthalmol 98:617, 1984.

Dark AJ, Streeten BW: Preinvasive carcinoma of the cornea and conjunctiva. Br J Ophthalmol 64:506, 1980.

Frazier PD, Wong VG: Cystinosis. Histologic and crystallographic examination of crystals in eye tissues. Arch Ophthalmol 80:87, 1968.

Glass R, Scheie HG, Yanoff M: Conjunctival amyloidosis arising from a plasmacytoma. Ann Ophthalmol 3:823, 1971.

Hanna C, Fraunfelder FT, Sanchez J: Ultrastructural study of argyrosis of the cornea and conjunctiva. Arch Ophthalmol 92:18, 1974.

Hogan MJ, Alvarado J: Pterygium and pinguecula: electron microscopic study. Arch Ophthalmol 78:174, 1967.

Kanai A, Polack FM: Histologic and electron microscopic studies of ligneous conjunctivitis. Am J Ophthalmol 72:909, 1972.

Lamping KA, et al: Oxyphil cell adenomas. Three case reports. Arch Ophthalmol 102:263, 1984.

Sandstrom I: Neonatal conjunctivitis caused by *Chlamydia trachomatis*. Acta Otolaryngol 407:67, 1984.

Wexler SA, Wallow IHL: Squamous cell carcinoma of the conjunctiva presenting with extraocular extension. Arch Ophthalmol 103:1175, 1985.

Yanoff M: Hereditary benign intraepithelial dyskeratosis. Arch Ophthalmol 79:291, 1968.

Yanoff M, Scheie HG: Argyrosis of the conjunctiva and lacrimal sac. Arch Ophthalmol 72:57, 1964.

CORNEA AND SCLERA 8

The cornea is one of the most unusual structures in the body in that it has no blood vessels and is crystal clear. Any pathological lesions, therefore, are seen easily as an opacification within the cornea. Numerous congenital abnormalities may involve the cornea. The defects range from complete absence of the cornea, to irregularities in the size or shape of the cornea, to congenital opacifications. Opacifications of the cornea may be present as isolated findings, e.g., a corneal keloid, or may be associated with systemic abnormalities, e.g., in cystinosis. In addition, corneal abnormalities may be associated with other ocular anomalies, especially those of the iris, lens, and anterior chamber angle, e.g., in Peters' anomaly and in Rieger's syndrome.

Inflammations commonly involve the cornea and can be broadly divided into two major types: nonulcerative and ulcerative. Both types may be caused by infectious or noninfectious agents. Inflammations generally affect the central cornea or the peripheral cornea. Following inflammation, numerous sequelae may occur which can result in decreased vision.

Degenerations, i.e., lesions that are secondary to previous disease, often involve the cornea. The degenerations may primarily affect the epithelium, e.g., recurrent erosion, or the stroma, e.g., arcus senilis.

Dystrophies are primary, usually inherited, bilateral disorders that have approximately equal involvement affecting both corneas. The dystrophy may affect the epithelium, e.g., in Meesmann's dystrophy; or Bowman's membrane, e.g., in Reis–Bücklers' dystrophy. Alternatively, the stroma (e.g., in granular dystrophy) or the endothelium (e.g., in cornea guttata) may be affected. Each dystrophy tends to have easily and readily identifiable clinical and histopathological characteristics. In addition to the primary corneal dystrophies, systemic disease (often metabolic and inherited, e.g., the acid mucopolysaccharidoses) may involve the cornea secondarily.

Because of the clarity of the cornea, deposition of pigment is seen easily. Many different types of pigment may be deposited in the cornea. The pigment may arise from local deposition, e.g., from epinephrine drops used in the treatment of glaucoma, or as part of a systemic disease, e.g., copper in the Kayser–Fleischer ring in Wilson's disease (hepatolenticular degeneration).

The sclera is composed of densely packed collagen and is relatively avascular, hence the white color seen clinically. It may be involved in congenital anomalies (e.g., in ochronosis), in inflammations (e.g., in scleritis) and in tumors (e.g., in episcleral osseous choristoma). Some of the more common and important scleral entities will be illustrated.

Fig. 8.1 CONGENITAL DEFECTS

Absence of cornea
Abnormalities of size
Microcornea (<11 mm in greatest diameter)
Megalocornea (>13 mm in greatest diameter)
Keratoglobus

Abberations of curvature
Astigmatism
Cornea plana
Keratoconus

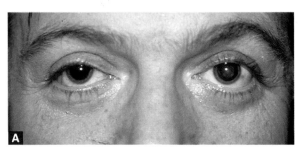

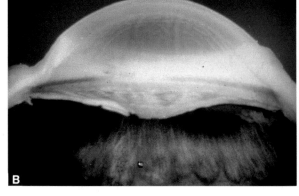

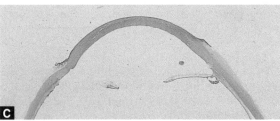

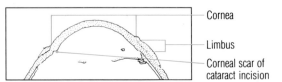

— Cornea

— Limbus

— Corneal scar of cataract incision

Fig. 8.2 Abnormalities of Size. A The patient has bilateral megalocornea, as do other male members of his family. The patient died from metastatic renal cell carcinoma, and the eyes were obtained at autopsy. **B** Gross examination shows an enlarged cornea and a very deep anterior chamber. **C** Histologic section shows that the cornea itself is of about normal diameter, but the limbal region is enlarged and slightly thicker than normal. The patient had had a cataract extraction and a peripheral iridectomy.

Fig. 8.3 CONGENITAL DEFECTS: CORNEAL OPACITIES

Anterior embryotoxon (arcus juvenilis)
Congenital leukomas (corneal keloids)
Central corneal dysgenesis
Peters' anomaly
Localized posterior keratoconus

Peripheral corneal and iris dysgenesis
Posterior embryotoxon (Axenfeld's syndrome)
Rieger's syndrome
Sclerocornea
**Limbal dermoids (may be associated
    with Goldenhar's syndrome)**

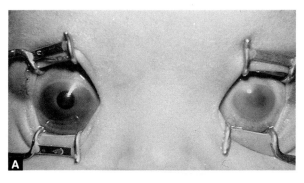

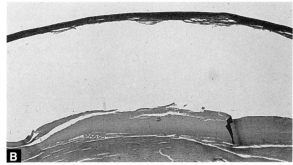

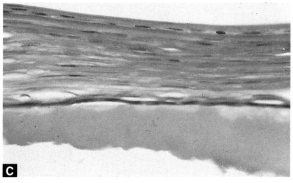

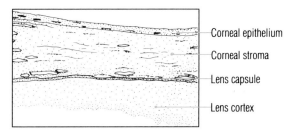

Corneal epithelium
Corneal stroma
Lens capsule
Lens cortex

Fig. 8.4 Peters' Anomaly. A The right eye shows an enlarged cornea, secondary to glaucoma. The left eye shows a small cornea as part of the anomalous affliction. **B** Histologic section shows considerable corneal thinning centrally. The space between the cornea and the lens material is artifactitious and secondary to shrinkage of the lens cortex during processing of the eye. **C** Increased magnification shows lens material attached to the posterior cornea. Centrally, no endothelium, Descemet's membrane, or Bowman's membrane are present. Lens capsule lines the posterior surface of the cornea. (**B, C,** PAS; case reported in Scheie HG and Yanoff M: Arch Ophthalmol 87:525, 1972.)

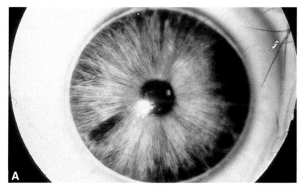

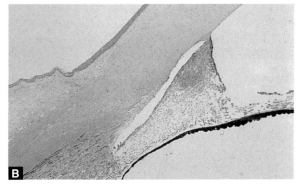

Fig. 8.5 Axenfeld's Syndrome (Posterior Embryotoxon). A Schwalbe's line is anteriorly displaced 360°. **B** Histologic section of another case shows an iris process attached to the anteriorly displaced Schwalbe's ring. (**A,** courtesy of Dr. WC Frayer; from *Ocular Pathology*, 2nd edn, by M Yanoff and BS Fine; **B,** courtesy of Dr. RY Foos.)

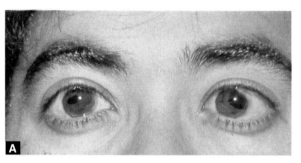

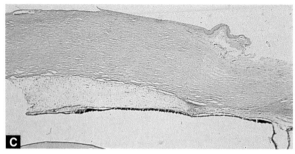

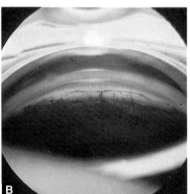

Fig. 8.6 Rieger's Syndrome. A The patient has numerous iris abnormalities and bilateral glaucoma. Note the hypertelorism. **B** The patient's daughter has similar abnormalities. Note the iris processes attached to an anteriorly displaced Schwalbe's line (anterior embryotoxon). **C** Histologic section of an eye from another patient shows an anteriorly displaced Schwalbe's ring. A diffuse abnormality of the iris stroma is present. (**A**, **B** courtesy of Dr. HG Scheie; **A**, from *Ocular Pathology*, 2nd edn, by M Yanoff and BS Fine.)

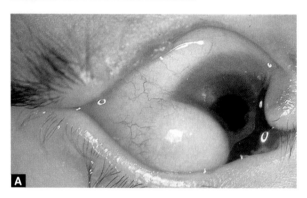

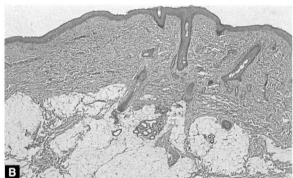

Fig. 8.7 Goldenhar's Syndrome. A The patient has bilateral, temporal limbal dermoids and a coloboma of this right upper lid. **B** The dermoid is composed of epidermis, dermis, epidermal appendages, and adipose tissue. (**A** courtesy of Dr. JA Katowitz; from *Ocular Pathology*, 2nd edn, by M Yanoff and BS Fine.)

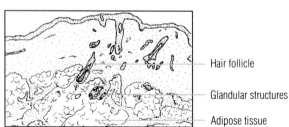

Hair follicle

Glandular structures

Adipose tissue

Fig. 8.8 NONULCERATIVE INFLAMMATIONS

Punctate epithelial keratitis
Subepithelial keratitis
Epidemic keratoconjunctivitis
Trachoma
Leprosy
Superior limbal keratoconjunctivitis

Stromal (interstitial) keratitis
Syphilis
Tuberculosis
Sarcoidosis
Onchocerciasis
Protozoal
Leishmaniasis
Trypanosomiasis

Viral
Herpes simplex
Herpes zoster
Cogan's syndrome
Hodgkin's disease
Mycosis fungoides
Lymphogranuloma venereum
Hypoparathyroidism

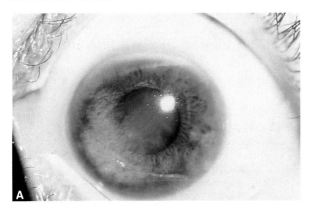

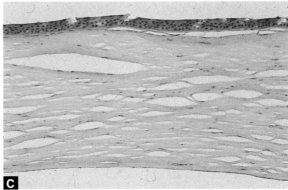

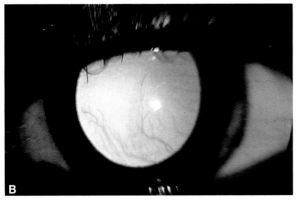

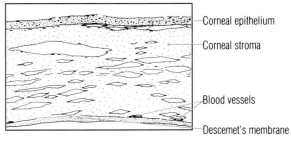

Fig. 8.9 Syphilis. A The cornea shows a range of opacification from a cloud-like nebula to a moderately dense macula to a very dense white leukoma. **B** In another case, ghost vessels are easily seen by retroillumination. **C** The vessels are deep in the corneal stroma, just anterior to Descemet's membrane. (**A**, courtesy of Dr. WC Frayer; **B** from *Ocular Pathology*, 2nd edn, by M Yanoff and BS Fine.)

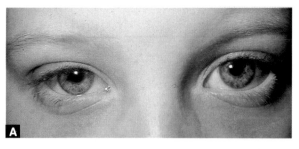

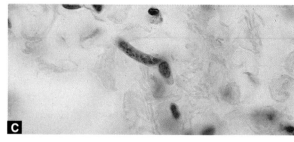

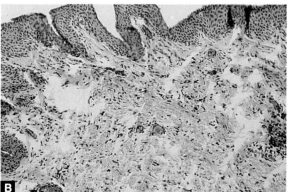

Fig. 8.10 Onchocerciasis. A This young girl had just returned from Africa. She had conjunctival injection and small corneal opacities at all levels. During examination at the slit lamp, a tiny thread-like worm was noted in the aqueous. B Histologic section of a conjunctival biopsy shows a chronic nongranulomatous inflammation and a tiny segment of the worm in the deep substantia propria; this is shown under higher magnification in C. (Case reported in Scheie HG et al: Ann Ophthalmol 3:697, 1971.)

Fig. 8.11 ULCERATIVE INFLAMMATIONS

Peripheral	Central
Marginal (catarrhal) ulcer	Bacterial
Phlyctenular ulcer	Viral
Ring ulcer	Mycotic
Ring abscess	

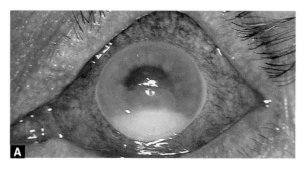

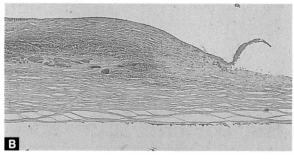

Fig. 8.12 Central Corneal Ulcer. A Note central ulcer and reactive, large hypopyon. B The right-hand side of the picture shows ulceration. The corneal stroma is infiltrated with polymorphonuclear leukocytes and large, amorphous, purple collections of material. Special stain of the purple areas showed a collection of many gram positive bacteria. (A, courtesy of Dr. HG Scheie.)

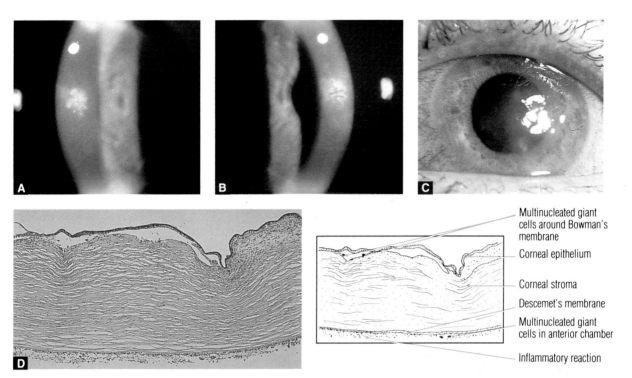

Multinucleated giant
cells around Bowman's
membrane

Corneal epithelium

Corneal stroma

Descemet's membrane

Multinucleated giant
cells in anterior chamber

Inflammatory reaction

Fig. 8.13   Herpes Simplex. A Typical dendritic ulcer is present in the central cornea, also shown with Rose Bengal in **B**. Note the characteristic terminal bulbs on the ulcer. **C** The patient had bullous keratopathy following long-standing herpes simplex keratitis (metaherpetic phase). **D** Histologic section shows a large, corneal epithelial bleb. Note the inflammatory reaction in the anterior chamber. Multinucleated giant cells are present in the region of Bowman's membrane and in the anterior chamber exudate. (**A** courtesy of Dr. HG Scheie; **D**, from *Ocular Pathology,* 2nd edn, by M Yanoff and BS Fine.)

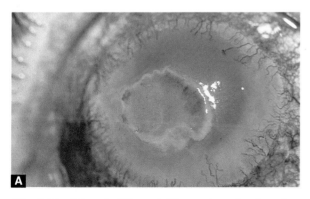

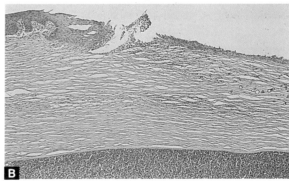

Fig. 8.14   Mycotic Ulcer. A The patient developed a central corneal ulcer that was caused by a pigmented fungus. **B** Histologic section of another case shows ulceration of the corneal epithelium, infiltration of the corneal stroma by polymorphonuclear leukocytes and large fungal elements. A hypopyon, consisting of polymorphonuclear leukocytes and cellular debris, is seen in the anterior chamber. Often fungal ulcers have satellite corneal lesions and a hypopyon.

Fig. 8.15 SEQUELAE OF INFLAMMATION

Descemetocele	Staphyloma	Adherent leukoma
Ectasia	Cicatrization	Vascularization

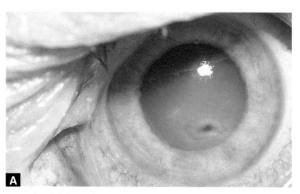

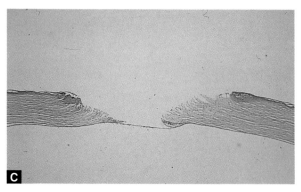

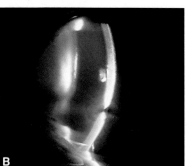

Fig. 8.16 Descemetocele. A and **B** show the clinical appearance of a descemetocele. **C** Histologic section of another case shows central loss of all corneal substance except Descemet's membrane. (**A** and **B** courtesy of Dr. IM Raber; **C**, PAS, from *Ocular Pathology*, 2nd edn, by M Yanoff and BS Fine.)

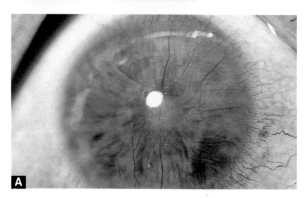

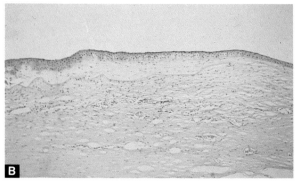

Fig. 8.17 Corneal Vascularization. A The corneal stroma is vascularized by large trunk vessels. **B** Corneal epithelial edema and stromal inflammation, scarring, and vascularization are present. A fibrotic scar (degenerative pannus) is seen between Bowman's membrane and the epithelium.

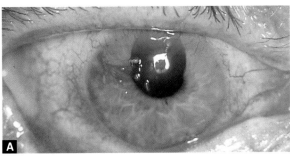

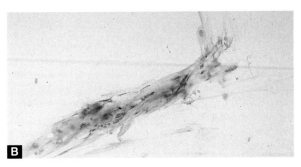

Fig. 8.19   Filamentary Keratitis. A Numerous filaments in the form of ropy secretions are present on the cornea, mainly superiorly. **B** Histologic section shows that the filaments are composed of epithelial cells and mucinous material. (**B**, from *Ocular Pathology*, 2nd edn, by M Yanoff and BS Fine.)

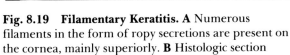

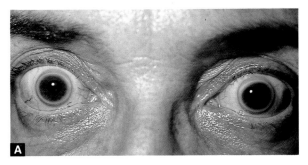

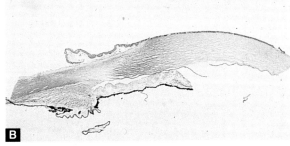

Fig. 8.21   Arcus Senilis. A A white ring is in the peripheral cornea of each eye. The ring is separated from the limbus by a typical tiny clear zone. **B** Histologic section shows that the lipid is concentrated in the anterior and posterior stroma as two red triangles, apex to apex, with the bases being Bowman's membrane and Descemet's membrane, both of which are infiltrated heavily by fat, as is the sclera. (**B**, oil red-O.)

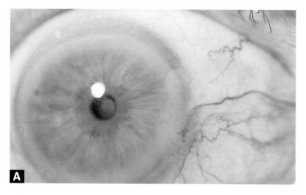

A

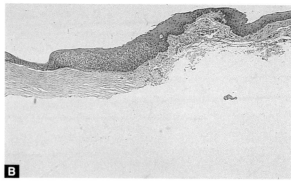

B

Fig. 8.22   Pterygium. A The nasal limbal conjunctiva and the contiguous cornea are involved by a vascularized lesion, a pterygium. **B** Histologic section shows basophilic degeneration of the substantia propria of the conjunctiva (identical to that seen in a pinguecula) toward the right and invasion of the cornea with destruction of Bowman's membrane toward the left. It is the invasion of the cornea that distinguishes a pterygium from a pinguecula (see Fig. 7.22).

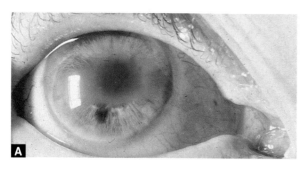

A

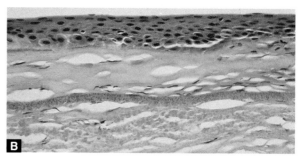

B

Fig. 8.23   Band Keratopathy. A Clinical appearance of the band occupying the central, horizontal zone of the cornea and typically sparing the most peripheral clear cornea. **B** A fibrous pannus is present between the epithelium and a calcified Bowman's membrane. Some deposit also is present in the anterior corneal stroma.

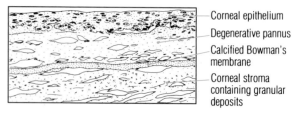

— Corneal epithelium
— Degenerative pannus
— Calcified Bowman's membrane
— Corneal stroma containing granular deposits

Fig. 8.24 DYSTROPHIES

Epithelial
Heredofamilial—primary
Meesmann's (Stocker–Holt)
Dot (microcystoid), fingerprint, and
    map (geographic) patterns
Heredofamilial—systemic
Fabry's disease

Bowman's membrane
Reis–Bückler's dystrophy

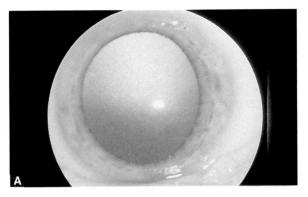

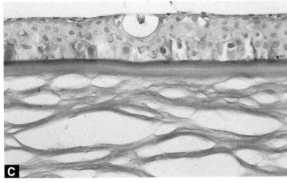

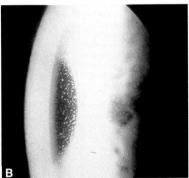

Fig. 8.25   Meesmann's Dystrophy. A and B show tiny, fine, punctate, clear vacuoles within the corneal epithelium. C Histologic section shows an intraepithelial cyst that contains debris. (B, from *Ocular Pathology*, 2nd edn, by M Yanoff and BS Fine; C, PAS; case reported in Fine BS, et al: Am J Ophthalmol 86:833, 1977.)

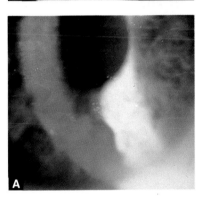

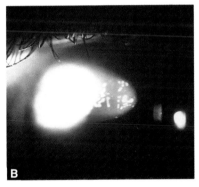

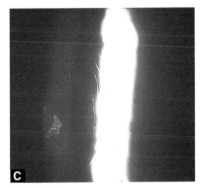

Fig. 8.26   Dot, Fingerprint, and Map Patterns. A The dot pattern is shown in the lower central cornea. A map pattern is seen above and to the left of the dot pattern. B The dot pattern resembles "putty" within the epithelium. C The fingerprint pattern, best seen with indirect lighting, is clearly shown. (B, courtesy of Dr. WC Frayer.)

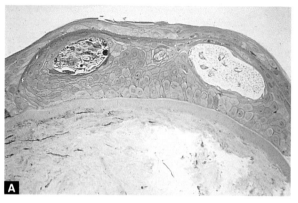

A

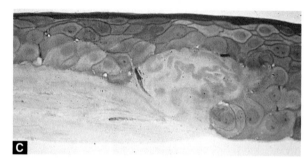

C

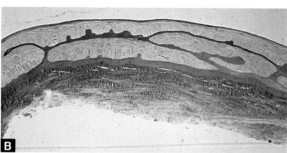

B

Fig. 8.27   Dot, Fingerprint, and Map Patterns. A Histologic section shows that the dot pattern is caused by cysts that contain desquamating surface epithelial cells. **B** The fingerprint pattern is caused by extensive, aberrant production of basement membrane material within the epithelium. **C** The map pattern is caused by accumulated subepithelial basement membrane and collagenous tissue that resembles a subepithelial fibrous plaque. (**A**, **B**, PD; from *Ocular Pathology*, 2nd edn, by M Yanoff and BS Fine; **C**, PD; cases reported in Rodriques MM, et al: Arch Ophthalmol 92:475, 1974.)

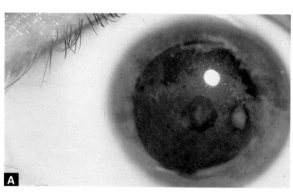

A

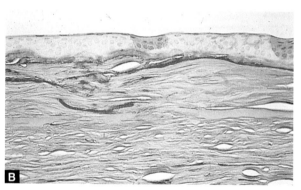

B

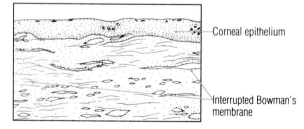

Corneal epithelium

Interrupted Bowman's membrane

Fig. 8.28   Reis–Bücklers' Dystrophy. A The characteristic, corneal, honeycombed pattern is apparent. **B** Histologic section shows disruption of Bowman's membrane by fibrous tissue, along with a fibrous plaque between Bowman's membrane and the epithelium. (**B**, trichrome.)

Fig. 8.29 STROMAL DYSTROPHIES

Heredofamilial—primary
Granular
Macular
Lattice
Congenital hereditary stromal dystrophy
Hereditary fleck dystrophy
Central stromal crystalline
 corneal dystrophy (Schnyder)

Heredofamilial—systemic
Mucopolysaccharidoses
Mucolipidoses
Sphingolipidoses
Ochronosis
Cystinosis
Hypergammaglobulinemia

Nonheredofamilial
Keratoconus
Keratoglobus
Pellucid marginal degeneration

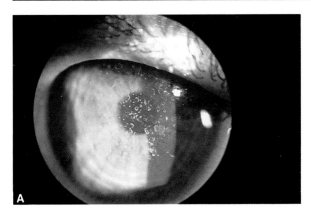

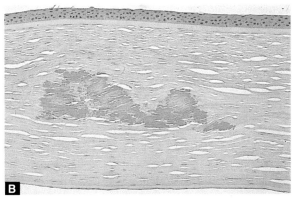

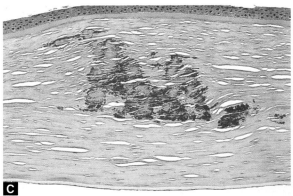

Fig. 8.30 Granular Dystrophy. A Clear cornea is present between the small, white, sharply outlined stromal granules. **B** Histologic section shows that the granules stain deeply with H&E and **C** stain red with the trichrome stain. The PAS stain and stains for acid mucopolysaccharides and amyloid are negative. The condition is inherited as an autosomal dominant trait.

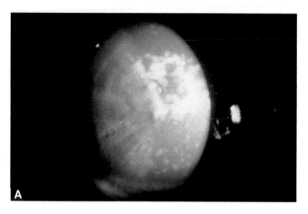

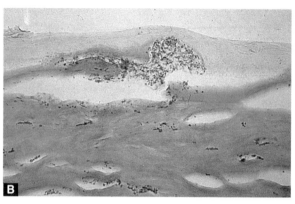

Fig. 8.31 Macular Dystrophy. A The corneal stroma between the opacities is cloudy. **B** Histologic section shows that keratocytes and vacuolated cells beneath the epithelium are filled with acid mucopoly-saccharide. In this condition, the trichrome stain and stains for amyloid are negative, but the PAS stain is positive. The condition is inherited as an autosomal recessive trait. (**B**, AMP.)

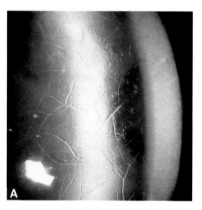

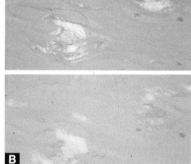

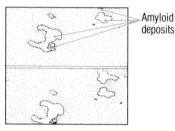

Amyloid deposits

Fig. 8.32 Lattice Dystrophy. A The lattice network is apparent in the corneal stroma. **B** Histologic section shows the positive staining with Congo red and positive birefringence. The color of the birefringence changes as the polarizer is moved 90°. Stains for acid mucopolysaccharides are negative, whereas the trichrome and PAS stains are positive. The condition is inherited as an autosomal dominant trait. (**A**, courtesy of Dr. JH Krachmer; **B**, Congo red, polarized; **A**, **B**, from *Ocular Pathology*, 2nd edn, by M Yanoff and BS Fine.)

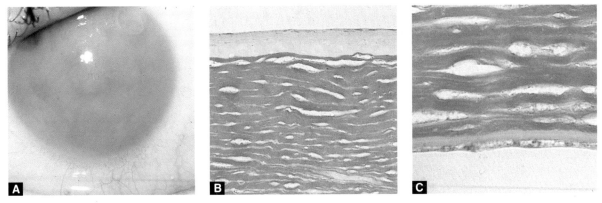

Fig. 8.33 Acid Mucopolysaccharidoses. A The cornea is diffusely clouded in a case of Hurler–Scheie syndrome. **B** Histologic section of a case of Maroteaux–Lamy syndrome shows acid mucopolysaccharides deposited in epithelial cells, stromal keratocytes, and **C** in endothelial cells. (**B & C**, AMP; **A**, case courtesy of Dr. HG Scheie; **B**, **C**, case courtesy of Dr. GOS Naumann.)

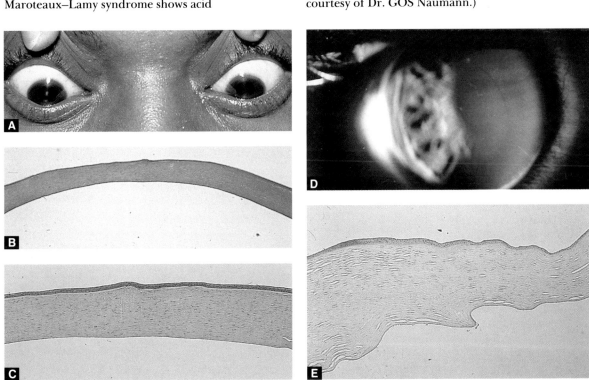

Fig. 8.34 Keratoconus. A When the patient looks down, the cone in each eye causes the lower lids to bulge (Munson's sign). **B** Histologic section shows the central thinning of the cornea. **C** Increased magnification of the central cone shows stromal scarring and breaks in Bowman's membrane. **D** A brown, Fleischer ring is noted in the cornea, at the level of the epithelium seen in the blue light. **E** Histologic section shows that the ring is caused by a deposition of iron in the corneal epithelium. Note the typical thinning of the cornea in the region of the cone to the right of the iron deposition. (**B**, PAS; **E**, Perl's stain.)

Fig. 8.35 ENDOTHELIAL DYSTROPHIES

Cornea guttata (Fuchs)   Congenital hereditary endothelial dystrophy
Posterior polymorphous dystrophy   Nonguttate corneal endothelial degeneration

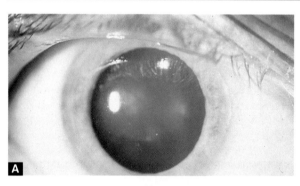

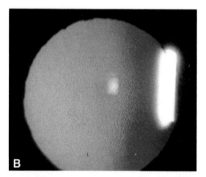

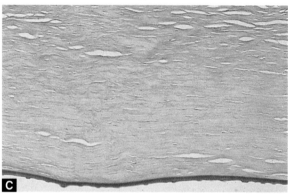

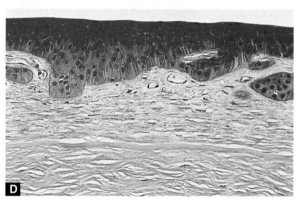

Fig. 8.36 Cornea Guttata. A The cornea shows central thickening and haze. **B** The characteristic appearance of cornea guttata is shown in the fundus reflex. **C** Typical, wart-like bumps are present on Descemet's membrane. The primary endothelial defect leads to secondary epithelial and stromal edema and degeneration. The edema may spread between and under the epithelial cells, resulting in bleb formation (bullous keratopathy). **D** Fibrous tissue may proliferate between the epithelium and Bowman's membrane, forming a degenerative pannus. (**B**, from *Ocular Pathology*, 2nd edn, by M Yanoff and BS Fine; **C**, PAS; **D**, trichrome.)

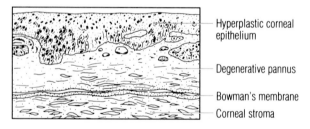

Hyperplastic corneal epithelium

Degenerative pannus

Bowman's membrane

Corneal stroma

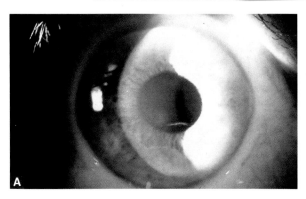 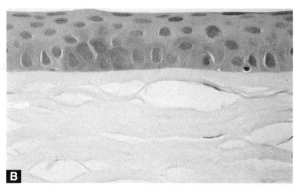

Fig. 8.38 Hudson–Stahli Line. A A horizontal brown line is seen just below the central cornea within the epithelium. **B** Histologic section shows that the line is caused by iron deposition within the epithelium. The other iron lines (Fleischer, Stocker, and Ferry) have a similar histologic appearance. (**B**, Perl's stain.)

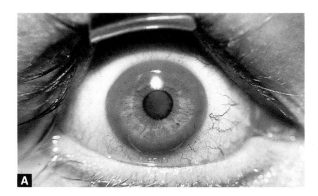 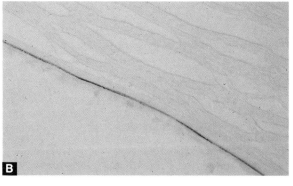

Fig. 8.39 Kayser–Fleischer Ring. A The deposition of copper in Descemet's membrane peripherally causes a brown color that obstructs the view of the underlying iris, especially superiorly. A "sunflower" cataract is seen in the lens. **B** An unstained histologic section shows the deposition of copper in the inner portion of Descemet's membrane. A similar deposition of copper in the inner portion of the lens capsule centrally, both anteriorly and posteriorly, results in the sunflower cataract. (**A**, courtesy of Dr. MOM Tso; case in **A** and **B** reported in Tso MOM et al, Am J Ophthalmol 79:479, 1975.)

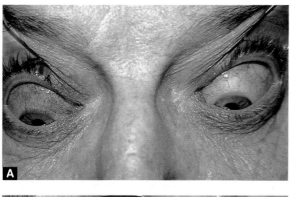

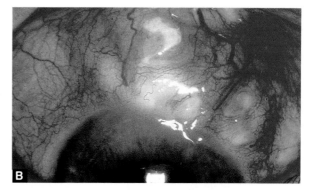

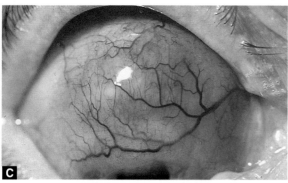

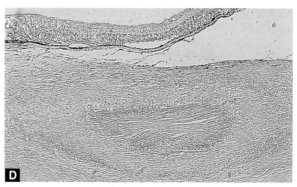

Fig. 8.41   Scleritis. Scleritis can go on to **A** thickening (brawny scleritis) and **B** necrosis. **C** Healing of the necrotic area leads to scleromalacia perforans. **D** Histologic section shows a zonal, granulomatous reaction around necrotic scleral collagen. (**D**, case presented by Dr. IW McLean at the 1973 AFIP Alumni meeting.)

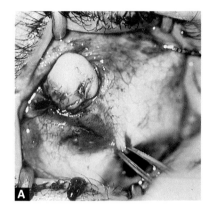

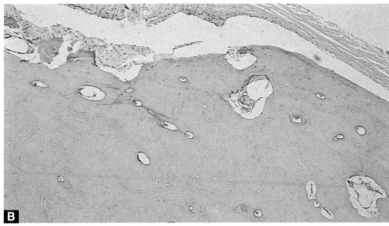

Fig. 8.42 Episcleral Osseous Choristoma. A The tumor, exposed at surgery, is located in its characteristic position, superotemporally. **B** Histologic section shows compact bone. (**B,** case reported in Ortiz JM and Yanoff M: Br J Ophthalmol 63:173, 1979.)

Bibliography

Cogan DG, Kuwabara T: Arcus senilis. Its pathology and histochemistry. Arch Ophthalmol 61:353, 1959.

Contreras F, Pereda J: Congenital syphilis of the eye with lens involvement. Arch Ophthalmol 96:1052, 1978.

Fine BS, Yanoff M, Pitts E, Slaughter FD: Meesmann's epithelial dystrophy of the cornea. Report of two families with discussion of the pathogenesis of the characteristic lesion. Am J Ophthalmol 83:633, 1977.

Kivlin JD, Fineman RM, Crandall AS, Olson RJ: Peters' anomaly as a consequence of genetic and nongenetic syndromes. Arch Ophthalmol 104:61, 1986.

Klintworth GK: Chronic actinic keratopathy—a condition associated with conjunctival elastosis (pinguecula) and typified by characteristic extracellular concretions. Am J Pathol 67:327, 1972.

Klintworth GK, Smith CF: Macular corneal dystrophy. Am J Pathol 89:167, 1977.

Krachmer JH, Feder RS, Belin MW: Keratoconus and related noninflammatory corneal thinning disorders. Review. Surv Ophthalmol 28:293, 1984.

Mansour AM, Wang F, Henkind P, Goldberg R, Shprintzen R: Ocular findings in the facioauriculovertebral sequence (Goldenhar–Gorlin syndrome). Am J Ophthalmol 100:555, 1985.

Meisler DM, Fine M: Recurrence of the clinical signs of lattice corneal dystrophy (Type I) in corneal transplants. Am J Ophthalmol 97:210, 1984.

Naumann G: Clearing of cornea after perforating keratoplasty in mucopolysaccharidosis type VI (Maroteaux–Lamy syndrome). N Engl J Med 312:995, 1985.

Ortiz JM, Yanoff M: Epipalpebral conjunctival osseous choristoma. Br J Ophthalmol 63:173, 1979.

Rao NA, Marak GE, Hidayat AA: Necrotizing scleritis. A clinico-pathologic study of 41 cases. Ophthalmology 92: 1542, 1985.

Rodriques MM, Fine BS, Laibson PR, Zimmerman LE: Disorders of the corneal epithelium—a clinicopathologic study of dot, geographic and fingerprint patterns. Arch Ophthalmol 92:475, 1974.

Rodriques MM, Gaster RN, Pratt MV: Unusual superficial confluent form of granular cornea dystrophy. Ophthalmology 90:1507, 1983.

Russell RG, Nasisse MP, Larsen HS, Rouse BT: Role of T-lymphocytes in the pathogenesis of herpetic stromal keratitis. Invest Ophthalmol Vis Sci 25:938, 1984.

Scheie HG, Shannon RE, Yanoff M: Onchocerciasis (ocular). Ann Ophthalmol 3:697, 1971.

Shields MB, Buckley E, Klintworth GK, Thresher R: Axenfeld–Rieger syndrome. A spectrum of developmental disorders. Review. Surv Ophthalmol 29:387, 1985.

Tso MOM, Fine BS, Thorpe HE: Kayser–Fleischer ring and associated cataract in Wilson's disease. Am J Ophthalmol 79:479, 1975.)

Zaidman GW, Geeraets R, Paylor RR, Ferry AP: The histopathology of filamentary keratitis. Arch Ophthalmol 103:1178, 1985.

UVEA 9

The uvea is composed of iris, ciliary body, and choroid. Congenital and developmental defects may involve any part of the uveal tract. The defects may be as simple as a persistent pupillary membrane or as complex as some of the colobomas of the choroid which contain contiguous orbital cystic structures. The uveal anomaly may be associated with systemic findings, such as in the oculocerebrorenal syndrome of Miller in which Wilms' tumor, genitourinary anomalies, and aniridia are found.

Inflammation of the uvea is quite common. The specific entities have been discussed in the appropriate chapters on nongranulomatous (Chapter 3) and granulomatous (Chapter 4) inflammations.

Systemic diseases often affect the uvea. Perhaps the most common association is with diabetes mellitus. In addition, juvenile xanthogranuloma (JXG) is found mainly in children under 6 months of age, characteristically involves the iris, and may cause a spontaneous hyphema. When confronted with an infant who has a spontaneous hyphema, one must consider JXG, retinoblastoma (iris neovascularization here can cause bleeding into the anterior chamber),

and trauma (histories are unreliable in infants and, although the parent may think the hemorrhage was spontaneous, it could have been caused by trauma).

Many atrophies and degenerations affect the uvea. Macular degeneration, one of the leading causes of blindness, is described separately in Chapter 11.

The uvea may be involved in a number of dystrophies. Most of these are inherited. Our knowledge of both the underlying causes and of the pathology of these entities is still in its infancy.

The most common primary malignant tumor of the eye is the malignant melanoma that is found in the choroid. Melanomas will be described separately with pigmented tumors of the eye (Chapter 17). Other tumors can arise from the pigment epithelium, from the mesenchymal tissue of the uvea, from the vascular tissue, and so forth. Some of the more important examples are shown below. In addition to primary tumors of the uvea, systemic tumors may involve the uvea secondarily, e.g., as metastases or in multifocal entities such as leukemias and lymphomas.

Fig. 9.1 CONGENITAL ABNORMALITIES

Persistent pupillary membrane (if minor, considered a normal finding)
Persistent tunica vasculosa lentis
Heterochromia iridis
Hematopoiesis (normal finding in infant)

Ectopic lacrimal gland
Hypoplasia of iris
Dysgenesis of cornea and iris
Coloboma
Cyst (see Fig. 2.14**B**)

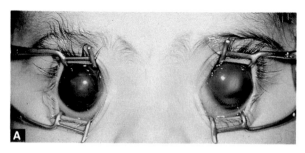

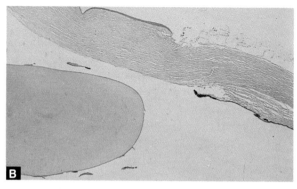

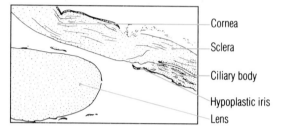

Fig. 9.2 Aniridia. **A** The child has bilateral aniridia and glaucoma. **B** A histologic section of another case shows that true aniridia is not present, but rather a marked hypoplasia of the iris is seen, as noted by the rudimentary iris. True aniridia does not exist; seen clinically, "apparent aniridia", is always found histologically to be hypoplasia (hypoiridia). The condition of apparent aniridia may be associated with glaucoma, as occured in **B** or with Wilms' tumor, which did not occur in this case. (**A**, courtesy of Dr. HG Scheie, from *Ocular Pathology*, 2nd edn, by M Yanoff and BS Fine.)

Cornea
Sclera
Ciliary body
Hypoplastic iris
Lens

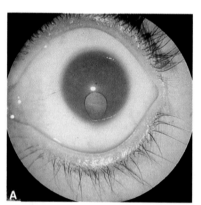

Fig. 9.3 Coloboma of Iris and Choroid **A** The patient is looking down, causing the light reflex to be centered in the choroidal coloboma, resulting in a white pupillary reflex (leukokoria). Note the small cornea and the microphthalmic eye. **B** A histologic section of another case of choroidal coloboma shows that the major defect is an absence of the retinal pigment epithelium. The overlying neural retina is atrophic and the underlying choroid is absent, so that the retina lies directly on the sclera. (**A**, courtesy of Dr. RC Lanciano, Jr.)

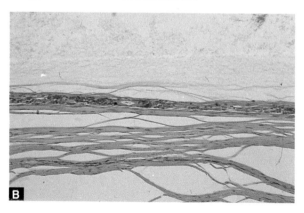

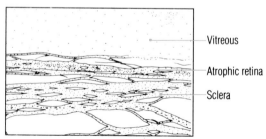

Vitreous
Atrophic retina
Sclera

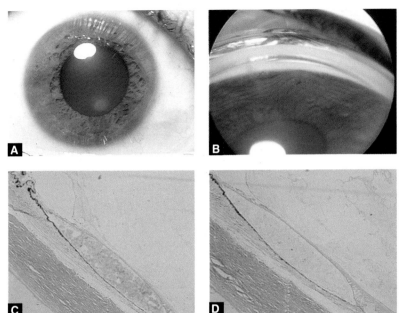

Fig. 9.4 Cysts of the Iris and Ciliary Body. **A** A bulge is present in the iris from the 9- to the 10-o'clock position. The stroma in this area is slightly atrophic. **B** Gonioscopic examination of the region clearly delineates the bulge that is caused by an underlying cyst of the pigment epithelium of the iris root. **C** A histologic section of another case shows a large cyst of the pars plana of the ciliary body. A special stain, which stains acid mucopolysaccharides blue, shows that the material within the cyst stains positively. **D** If the section is first digested with hyaluronidase and then stained as in **C**, the material is absent, demonstrating that the material in the cyst is hyaluronic acid.

Fig. 9.5 SYSTEMIC DISEASES

Diabetes mellitus	Homocystinuria	Histiocytosis X (Langerhans granulomatoses)
Vascular diseases	Amyloidosis	Collagen diseases
Cystinosis	Juvenile xanthogranuloma	Mucopolysaccharidoses

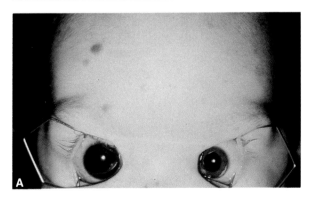

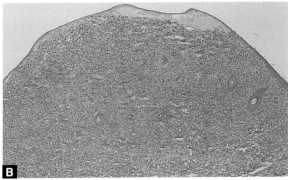

Fig. 9.6 Juvenile Xanthogranuloma (JXG). **A** The patient has multiple orange skin lesions (note the right side of the forehead), characteristic of JXG. Both eyes are involved. A spontaneous hyphema in the right eye had resulted in glaucoma and enlargement of the globe (buphthalmos). **B** Biopsy of the skin lesion shows that the dermis is largely replaced by histiocytes. The characteristic Touton giant cells were not found in these sections. However, the clinical picture and the histologic features were so characteristic that the diagnosis of JXG was not in doubt. (**B**, from *Ocular Pathology*, 2nd edn, by M Yanoff and BS Fine.)

Fig. 9.7 ATROPHIES AND DEGENERATIONS

Iris neovascularization (rubeosis iridis)
Choroidal folds

Fig. 9.8 DYSTROPHIES

Iridocorneal endothelial (ICE) syndrome
Iridoschisis
Regional choroidal dystrophies
Central areolar choroidal sclerosis
Serpiginous degeneration
Malignant myopia

Diffuse choroidal dystrophies
Diffuse choriocapillaris atrophy
Gyrate atrophy
Choroideremia

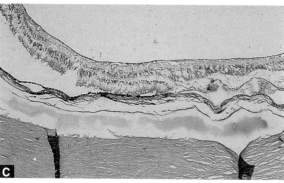

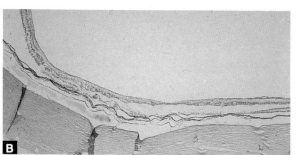

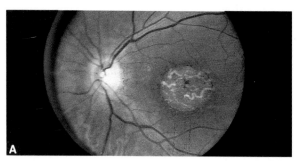

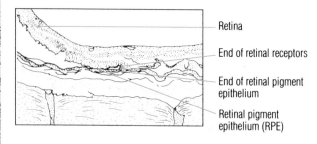

Retina

End of retinal receptors

End of retinal pigment
epithelium

Retinal pigment
epithelium (RPE)

Fig. 9.9 Central Areolar Choroidal Sclerosis. **A** The patient has bilateral, "punched-out" lesions of the macula. **B** A histologic section of another case shows loss of the pigment epithelium just temporal to the fovea (on the left side), shown under higher magnification in **C**. The photoreceptors are atrophic in the area of pigment epithelial loss. (**A**, courtesy of Dr. WE Benson, from *Ocular Pathology*, 2nd edn, by M Yanoff and BS Fine; **B**, **C** , presented by Dr. AP Ferry at the Eastern Ophthalmic Pathology Society in 1969 and also reported in Ferry AP et al: Arch Ophthalmol 88:39, 1972.)

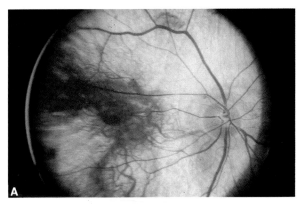

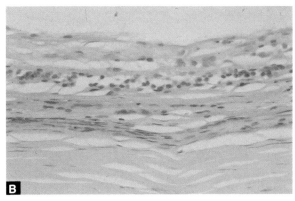

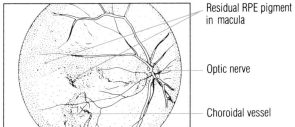

Residual RPE pigment
in macula

Optic nerve

Choroidal vessel

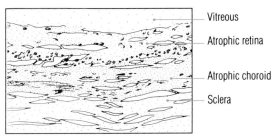

Vitreous

Atrophic retina

Atrophic choroid

Sclera

Fig. 9.10 Choroidermia. **A** Often in choroideremia a diffuse loss of the peripheral retinal pigment epithelium (RPE) occurs, leaving an island of RPE in the central macular region. **B** Histologic section of another case shows absence of RPE and atrophy of the overlying retina and underlying choroid. (**A**, courtesy of Dr. WE Benson, from *Ocular Pathology*, 2nd edn, by M Yanoff and BS Fine; **B**, case presented by Dr. WS Hunter at AOA-AFIP meeting in 1969.)

Fig. 9.11 TUMORS

Epithelial
Hypertrophy of retinal pigment epithelium (RPE)
Hyperplasia of RPE
Benign epithelioma (adenoma) of Fuchs
Muscular
Leiomyoma
Rhabdomyosarcoma
Vascular
Hemangioma

Osseous
Osseous choristoma
Melanoma (see Chapter 17)
Leukemias and lymphomas
Neural
Secondary neoplasms

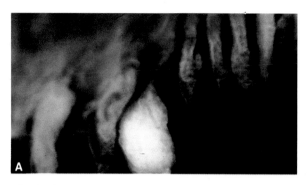

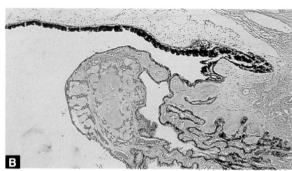

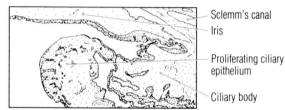

Fig. 9.12 Fuchs' Adenoma. **A** The lesion is seen grossly as a white tumor within the pars plicata of the ciliary body. **B** Histologic section shows a proliferation of nonpigmented ciliary epithelium that is elaborating considerable basement membrane material. (**A**, from *Ocular Pathology*, 2nd edn, by M Yanoff and BS Fine.)

Sclemm's canal
Iris

Proliferating ciliary epithelium

Ciliary body

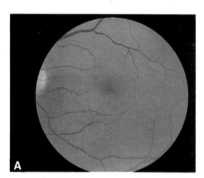

Fig. 9.13 Hemangioma. **A** An elevated lesion, which shows a characteristic orange color, is seen in the inferior, nasal macular region. **B** A histologic section of another case shows a total retinal detachment and an extensive hemangioma of the choroid in the macular area. **C** Increased magnification of the temporal edge of the hemangioma shows that it is blunted and well demarcated from the adjacent normal choroid to the left. **D** Similarly, the nasal edge of the hemangioma is blunted and easily demarcated from the adjacent choroid. This hemangioma was not associated with any systemic findings; in Sturge–Weber syndrome, the choroidal hemangioma is diffuse and not clearly demarcated from the adjacent choroid.

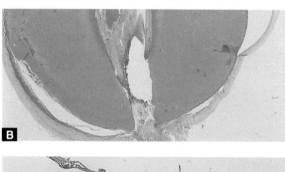

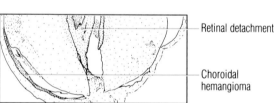

Retinal detachment

Choroidal hemangioma

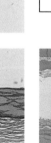

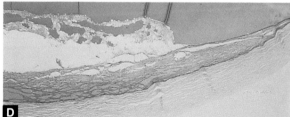

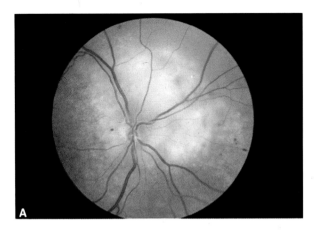

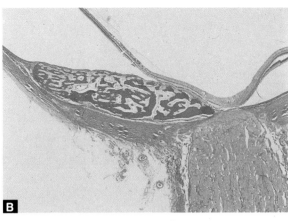

Fig. 9.14 Choroidal Osteoma. **A** The patient has an irregular, slightly elevated, yellow-white, juxta-papillary lesion. Ultrasound testing showed the characteristic features of bone in the choroid. **B** A histologic section of another case shows that the choroid is replaced by mature bone which contains marrow spaces. (**A,** courtesy of Dr. WE Benson, from *Ocular Pathology*, 2nd edn, by M Yanoff and BS Fine; **B**, case presented by Dr. RL Font in 1976 at the Eastern Ophthalmic Pathology Society.)

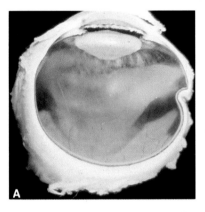

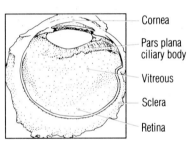

Cornea

Pars plana ciliary body

Vitreous

Sclera

Retina

Fig. 9.15 Reticulum Cell Sarcoma. **A** The gross specimen shows a cloudy and prominent vitreous body. The patient had been treated for posterior uveitis in both eyes for over a year when symptoms of a central nervous system disorder developed. **B** The vitreous body contains cells that show pleomorphism and hyperchromatic nuclei. The cells are quite abnormal and malignant. Although the cells in this entity are not reticulum cells but are lymphoblasts, the term reticulum cell sarcoma is still useful in conjuring up the clinical picture. (**A,** from *Ocular Pathology*, 2nd edn, by M Yanoff and BS Fine; case presented by Dr. M Yanoff in 1974 at Verhoeff Society Meeting.)

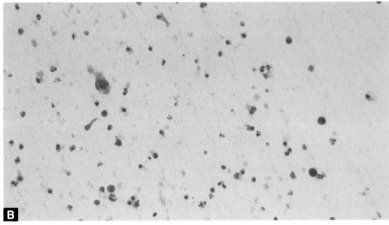

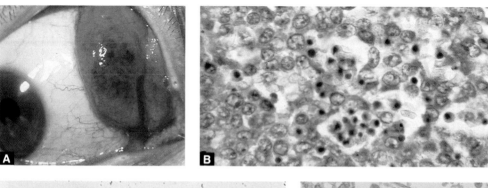

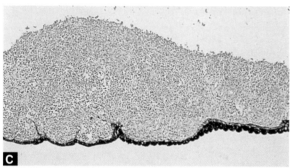

Fig. 9.16 Leukemia. **A** A patient presented with a large infiltrate of leukemic cells positioned nasally within the conjunctiva of the right eye, giving this characteristic clinical picture. Lesions such as this look quite similar to those caused by benign lymphoid hyperplasia or amyloidosis. **B** A biopsy of the lesion shows primitive, blastic leukocytes. **C** In another case, the iris is infiltrated by leukemic cells. A special stain (Lader stain) shows that some of the cells stain red, better seen when viewed under increased magnification in **D**. This red positivity is characteristic of myelogenous leukemic cells.

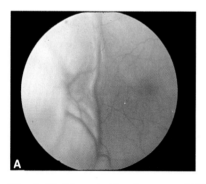

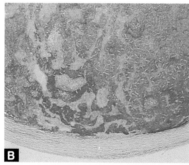

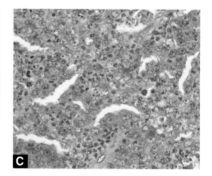

Fig. 9.17. Metastic Carcinoma. **A** The patient had an adenocarcinoma of the lung that metastasized to the eye. **B** A histologic section shows dark and light areas. The dark areas represent the cellular tumor, and the light areas represent stroma. Even under low magnification, a choroidal malignant melanoma can be ruled out because a melanoma does not have any stroma. **C** Increased magnification shows the malignant epithelial cells, many of which show mitotic figures. (**A**, from *Ocular Pathology*, 2nd edn, by M Yanoff and BS Fine.)

Bibliography

Alamanaseer IY, Kosova L, Pellettiere EV: Composite lymphoma with immunoblastic features and Langerhans cell granulomatosis (Histiocytosis X). Am J Clin Pathol 85:111, 1986.

Coburn A et al: Spontaneous intrastromal iris cyst. A case report with immunohistochemical and ultrastructural observations. Ophthalmology 92:1691, 1985.

Ferry AP, Llovera I, Shafer DM: Central areolar choroidal dystrophy. Arch Ophthalmol 88:39, 1972.

Gass JDM et al: Multifocal pigment epithelial detachments by reticulum cell sarcoma: a characteristic funduscopic picture. Retina 4:135, 1984.

Kincaid MC, Green WR: Ocular and orbital involvement in leukemia (Review). Surv Ophthalmol 27:211, 1983.

Lang GK et al: Ocular reticulum cell sarcoma. Clinicopathologic correlation of a case with multifocal lesions. Retina 5:79, 1985.

Nelson LB et al: Aniridia. A review. Surv Ophthalmol 28:621, 1984.

Rodriques MM et al: Choroideremia: a clinical, electron microscopic and biochemical report. Ophthalmology 91:873, 1984.

Trimble SN, Schatz H: Choroidal osteoma after intraocular inflammation. Am J Ophthalmol 96:759, 1983.

Waeltermann JM, Hettinger ME, Cibis GW: Congenital cysts of the iris stroma. Am J Ophthalmol 100:549, 1985.

Zimmerman LE: Ocular lesions of juvenile xanthogranuloma. Nevoxanthoendothelioma. Trans Am Acad Ophthalmol Otolaryngol 69:412, 1965.

LENS 10

The lens is unusual for a number of reasons. It has surface epithelium which grows inward at the equator; therefore, during its transformation into functional lens tissue, it has nowhere to shed. This causes the lens to become increasingly compacted with age. The compaction is often coupled with the deposition of yellow pigment. On the one hand, the presence of the yellow pigment and the compaction decrease the penetration of light and decrease vision; on the other hand, they preferentially filter out ultraviolet light and may help to protect the macular portion of the retina against light damage. Lens epithelial cells are quite reactive and participate in the formation of certain kinds of cataract but do not seem to have the ability to undergo neoplastic change, a characteristic that they share to some extent with the cells of the retinal pigment epithelium.

Many congenital abnormalities of the lens have been described. These range from very simple abnormalities, such as a Mittendorf dot, to very complex abnormalities that may be secondary to a metabolic defect, such as occur in galactosemia.

The capsule of the lens is a basement membrane that is secreted by the lens epithelium and is the thickest basement membrane in the body. The capsule may participate in ocular lesions such as true exfoliation and the exfoliation syndrome.

The epithelium may be damaged by a noxious stimulus, such as trauma or inflammation, and may then proliferate to form either an anterior or posterior subcapsular cataract (or both). Following trauma the epithelium may form abnormal lens cells that result in the development of Elschnig pearls, or may form a secondary thickening on the posterior lens capsule.

With aging, the cortex of the lens tends to become denatured and undergoes degeneration, forming globules of liquefied cortex that are called morgagnian globules. Materials, such as cholesterol may become deposited in the cortex. Also, fluid clefts (water clefts) may form. The process may continue to an extreme degree so that all of the cortex becomes liquefied and milky white, called a mature or morgagnian cataract. The fluid may escape through the intact lens capsule and result in a shrinking of the substance of the lens and a redundancy or folding of the capsule, called a hypermature cataract.

The nucleus of the lens, in contrast to the "soft" cortex, tends to be "hard". With aging, in addition to the accumulation of pigment, other substances such as calcium oxalate may be deposited. Cortical and nuclear cataracts may occur at any age, but tend to have two peaks; one peak under 10 years of age and caused mainly by congenital factors, and the other peak after 60 years of age, as a "normal" aging process.

Cataracts may be secondary to a variety of local and systemic abnormalities, as well as to metabolic diseases and trauma. Whatever the cause of the cataract, a number of complications may occur. Through a variety of mechanisms, the cataract may cause glaucoma or inflammation. An ectopic lens may arise due to a congenital (e.g., Marfan's syndrome) or acquired (e.g., traumatic subluxation or dislocation) condition.

Fig. 10.1 CONGENITAL ABNORMALITIES

Mittendorf dot
Aphakia
Duplication
Fleck cataract
Anterior polar cataract
Posterior polar cataract
Anterior lenticonus
Posterior lenticonus

Congenital cataract
Zonular
Sutural
Axial
Membranous
Filiform
Secondary to intrauterine
    infection

Galactosemia
Transient neonatal lens vacuoles

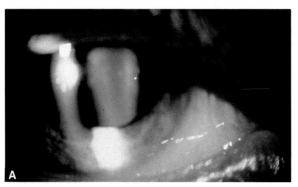

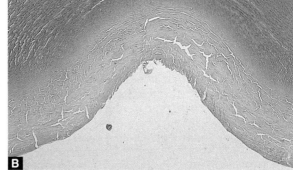

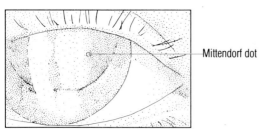

Mittendorf dot

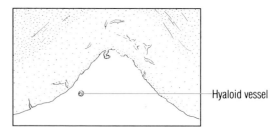

Hyaloid vessel

Fig. 10.2   Mittendorf Dot. A The hyaloid vessel remnant is seen as a small, white dot on the posterior surface of the lens, slightly nasal to the posterior pole of the lens. The attachment site is called a Mittendorf dot. **B** A histologic section shows the hyaloid vessel approaching the posterior surface of the lens. The posterior umbilication of the lens is an artifact of fixation, often seen in eyes obtained from infants and young children. (**A**, from *Ocular Pathology*, 2nd edn, by M Yanoff and BS Fine.)

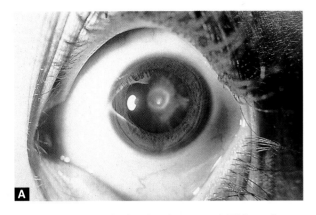

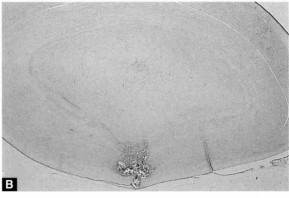

Fig. 10.3 Congenital Polar Cataract. A This patient had both anterior and posterior congenital polar cataracts. **B** Histologic section of another lens that contained a congenital posterior polar cataract shows degeneration of the posterior, subcapsular cortex.

Fig. 10.4 CAPSULE

General reactions	"True" exfoliation
Elasticity	Exfoliation syndrome
Thickening	
Thinning	
Rupture	

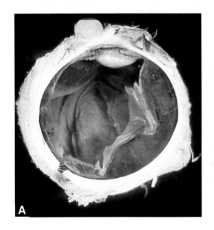

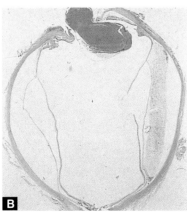

Fig. 10.5 Lens Capsule Elasticity. A This patient had developed bullous keratopathy, secondary to glaucoma. The cornea then became ulcerated and perforated, resulting in an expulsive choroidal hemorrhage. The eye was enucleated. Gross examination shows the massive choroidal hemorrhage and the lens protruding through the ruptured cornea. **B** A histologic section demonstrates the molding of the lens through the corneal opening. The lens capsule is intact.

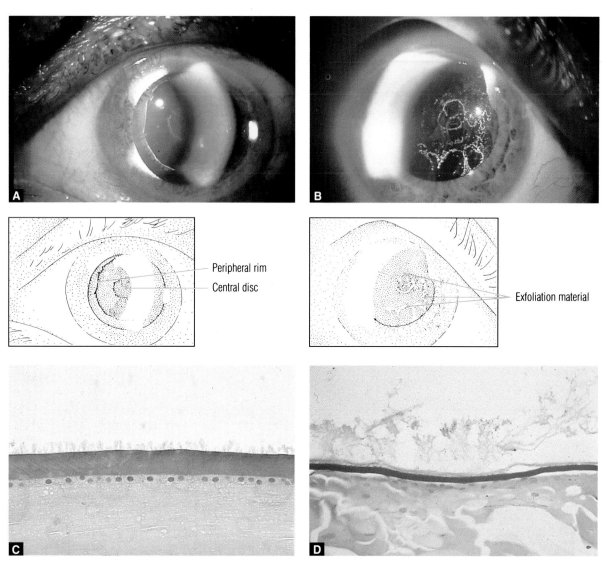

Fig. 10.6 Exfoliation Syndrome. A In this classic case of exfoliation syndrome, the anterior surface of the lens shows a central disc of exfoliation material, surrounded by a relatively clear area, which is in turn surrounded by a peripheral granular area. **B** Another patient who had mild exfoliation syndrome had an intracapsular cataract extraction. Over the years, the exfoliation material was deposited on the anterior face of the vitreous. **C** In the central disc area, the exfoliation material is deposited as small slivers that line up parallel to each other. **D** In the peripheral granular area, the material is in great abundance and has a thick, dendritic appearance. (**C, D**, PAS stain.)

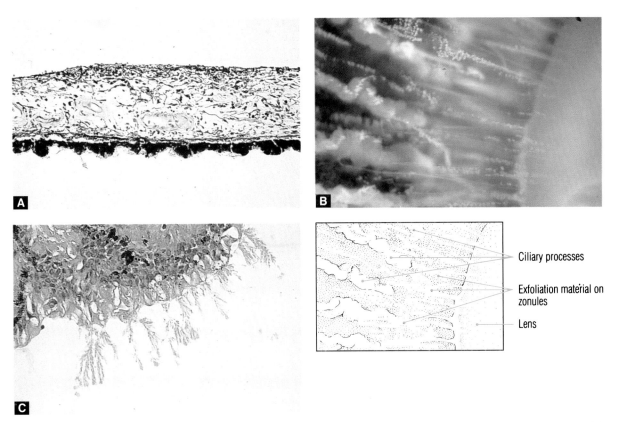

Ciliary processes

Exfoliation material on zonules

Lens

Fig. 10.7   Exfoliation Syndrome. A The exfoliation material deposits on the posterior surface of the iris, acting as a strut and causing the iris to have a sawtooth, posterior configuration. The deposited material often limits dilatation of the iris. The material also can be seen deposited on the zonular fibers of **B** the lens and **C** on the ciliary epithelium. (**B**, courtesy of Dr. RC Eagle Jr; **C**, PAS stain.)

Fig. 10.8 EPITHELIUM

Anterior subcapsular cataract   Elschnig pearls
Posterior subcapsular cataract   Degeneration and atrophy

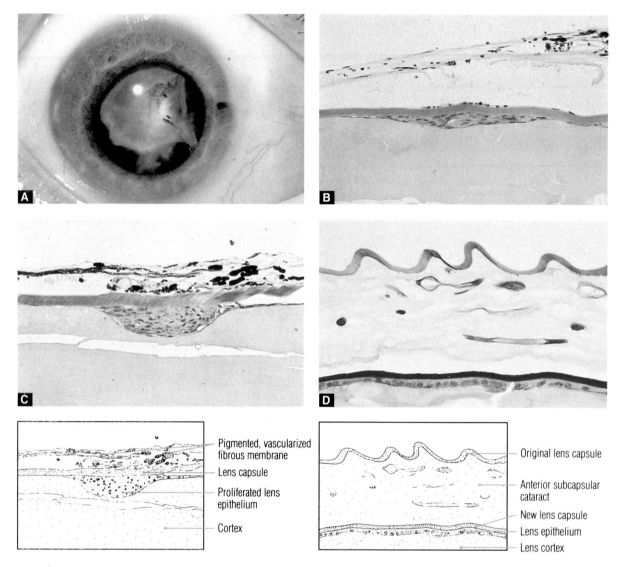

Fig.10.9 Anterior Subcapsular Cataract. A The patient developed an anterior subcapsular cataract some years after blunt trauma to this eye. **B** A histologic section of another case shows early proliferation of the lens epithelium underneath the capsule. **C** In another case, further proliferation of the lens epithelium has occurred along with fibroblastic metaplasia. **D** The proliferated epithelium has largely disappeared and has laid down collagen tissue. The original lens capsule is thrown into folds. The original lens epithelium has laid down a new lens capsule. (**B**, **C**, from *Ocular Pathology*, 2nd edn, by M Yanoff and BS Fine; **B**, **C**, and **D**, PAS stain.)

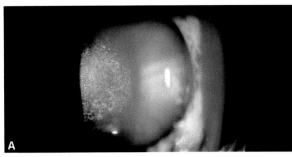

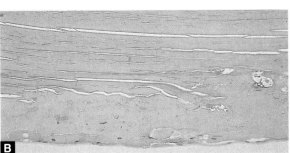

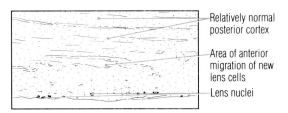

Relatively normal posterior cortex

Area of anterior migration of new lens cells

Lens nuclei

Fig. 10.10 Posterior Subcapsular Cataract. A The patient had been on long-term, systemic, steroid therapy following a renal transplant. Over the years, a cataract developed just anterior to the posterior surface of the lens. **B** A histologic section of another case shows migration of the lens epithelium to the posterior pole. Here the epithelial cells tend to form new, but abnormal, lens cells that migrate anteriorly into the posterior lens cortex. This lens was removed from a patient who had retinitis pigmentosa.

Fig. 10.11 CORTEX AND NUCLEUS

Cortex: "soft" cataract	Nucleus: "hard" cataract

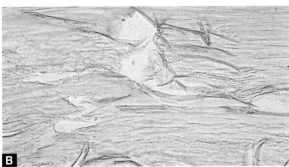

Fig. 10.12 Cholesterolosis Lentis. A The patient had glistening crystals in the cortex of both eyes. **B** Frozen sectioning of the removed lens shows clear areas. **C** Polarization of the clear areas demonstrates birefringent material, characteristic of cholesterol.

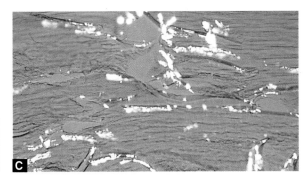

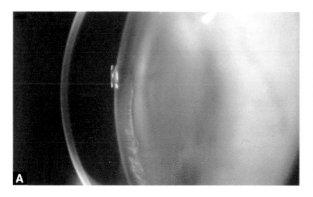

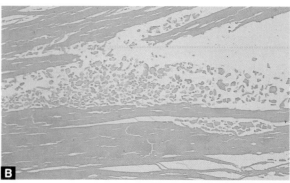

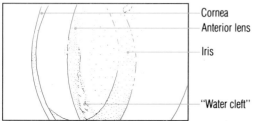

Cornea
Anterior lens
Iris

"Water cleft"

Fig. 10.13 Morgagnian Degeneration. A Slit lamp examination of the lens shows a "water cleft" that is composed of liquefied cortex in the form of morgagnian degeneration. **B** A histologic section of another case shows the morgagnian globules between fragmented cortical lens "fibers".

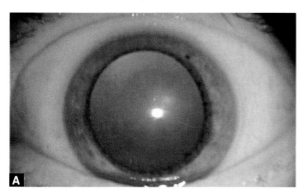

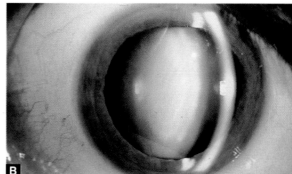

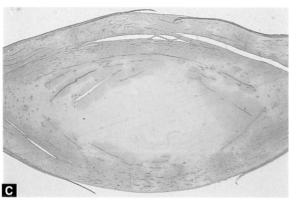

Fig. 10.14 Nuclear Cataract. A The red reflex shows the "oil droplet" effect of the nuclear cataract. **B** Slit lamp examination of another case shows the cataractous, yellow-pigmented nucleus. **C** A histologic section of another case shows the homogeneous nature of the compacted cells within the nuclear cataract. (**B**, from *Ocular Pathology*, 2nd edn, by M Yanoff and BS Fine.)

Fig. 10.15 SECONDARY CATARACTS

| Intraocular disease | Toxic | Endocrine and metabolic |

Fig. 10.16 COMPLICATIONS OF CATARACTS

Glaucoma
Mechanical
Phacolytic
Phacoanaphylactic
  endophthalmitis

Ectopic lens
Congenital with systemic diseases
Homocystinuria
Marfan's syndrome
Weill–Marchesani syndrome
Cutis hyperelastica (Ehlers–Danlos syndrome)
Proportional dwarfism
Oxycephaly
Crouzon's disease
Sprengel's deformity
Sturge–Weber syndrome

Congenital without systemic
  disease
Simple ectopic lens
Ectopic lens and pupil
Acquired ectopic lens
Nontraumatic
Traumatic

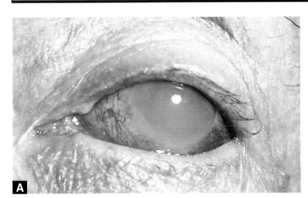

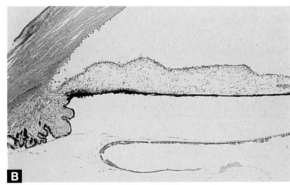

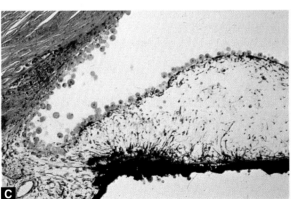

Fig. 10.17   Phacolytic Glaucoma. A The patient presented with signs and symptoms of acute closed-angle glaucoma. Chalky material was present in the anterior chamber. **B** A histologic section of another eye shows that no lens cortex is present within the lens. The liquefied cortex had "leaked out" through an intact capsule, resulting in a hypermature cataract. The lens material then was phagocytosed by macrophages that are present on the anterior surface of the iris and within the open angle of the anterior chamber. **C** Increased magnification of another section better shows the macrophages. The macrophages are swollen because of the ingested lens material.

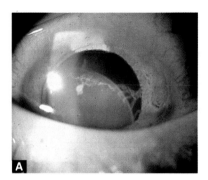

Fig. 10.18 Homocystinuria. A A fringe of white zonular remnants are present at the equator of the lens. These remnants tend to undulate slowly when the eye moves. The lens is subluxated inferonasally, the usual location in homocystinuria (in Marfan's syndrome it is most often subluxated superotemporally). **B** A histologic section of another case shows a thrombus in the greater arterial circle of the ciliary body. Patients who have homocystinuria are prone to thrombotic episodes, especially during or after general anesthesia. **C** A characteristic thick mantle of abnormal zonular material covers the pars plana of the ciliary body. (Case shown in **A** reported in Ramsey MS et al: Arch Ophthalmol 93:318, 1975; **C**, PAS stain.)

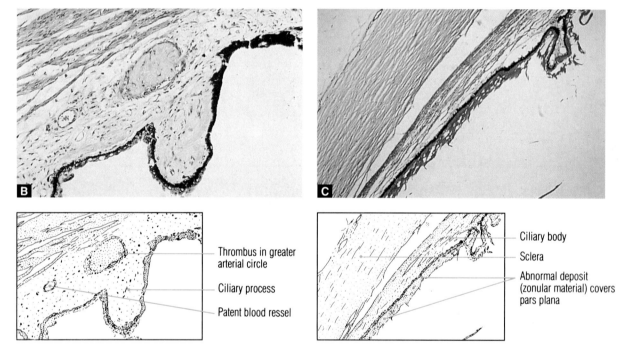

Thrombus in greater arterial circle

Ciliary process

Patent blood ressel

Ciliary body

Sclera

Abnormal deposit (zonular material) covers pars plana

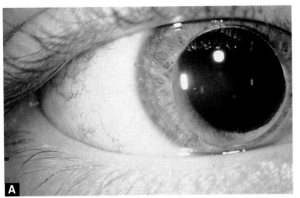

A

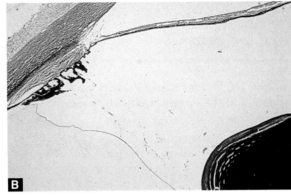

B

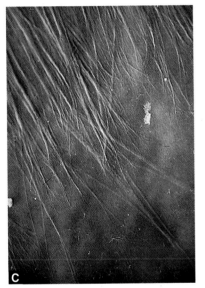

C

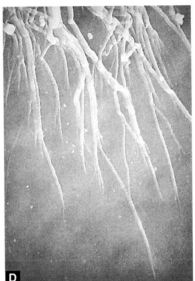

D

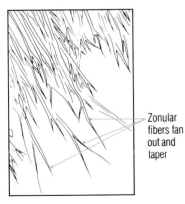

Zonular
fibers fan
out and
taper

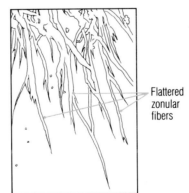

Flattered
zonular
fibers

Fig. 10.19 Marfan's Syndrome.
A The lens has dislocated into the anterior chamber. Actually, in Marfan's syndrome, the lens usually subluxates superotemporally in the posterior chamber rather than dislocating into the anterior chamber, (as has occurred here). Anterior dislocation is most common with homocystinuria. **B** A histologic section from an infant shows a relatively normal anterior segment. **C** Scanning electron microscopic examination of the lens from a normal individual shows the zonular fibers spread out over the anterior lens capsule. Note the fanning out and the tapering of the fibers. **D** The zonular fibers inserting into the anterior capsule in a patient with Marfan's syndrome show a flattening and a rapid attenuation of the fibers along with a lack of wide separation into a fan of filaments, probably representing a weakened attachment site. (**A**, courtesy of Dr. AC Wulc; **B**, reticulum stain; **C, D**, electron micrographs; case shown in **D** reported in Ramsey MS et al: Am J Ophthalmol 76:102, 1972.)

Bibliography

Chylack LT Jr: Mechanisms of senile cataract formation. Ophthalmology 91:596, 1984.

Chylack LT Jr, Ransil BJ, White O: Classification of human senile cataractous change by the American Cooperative Cataract Research Group (CCRG) method:III. The association of nuclear color (sclerosis) with extent of cataract formation, age, and visual acuity. Invest Ophthalmol Vis Sci 25:174, 1984.

Kozart, DM, Yanoff M: Intraocular pressure status in 100 consecutive patients with exfoliation syndrome. Ophthalmology 89:214, 1982.

Flach AJ, Peterson JS, Dolan BJ: Anterior subcapsular cataracts: a review of potential etiologies. Ann Ophthalmol 17:78, 1985.

Henkind P, Prose P: Anterior polar cataract: electron microscopic evidence of collagen. Am J Ophthalmol 63:768, 1967.

Nelson LB, Maumenee IH: Ectopic lentis (Review). Surv Ophthalmol 27:143, 1982.

Ramsey MS, Daitz LD, Beaton JW: Lens fringe in homocystinuria. Arch Ophthalmol 93:318, 1975.

Ramsey MS et al: The Marfan syndrome. A histopathologic study of ocular findings. Am J Ophthalmol 76:102, 1973.

Ramsey MS, Fine BS, Yanoff M: The ocular histopathology of homocystinuria. A light and electron microscopic study. Am J Ophthalmol 74:377, 1972.

Smith ME, Zimmerman LE: Contusive angle recession in phacolytic glaucoma. Arch Ophthalmol 74:799, 1965.

Streeten BW, Eshaghian J: Human posterior subcapsular cataract. A gross and flat preparation study. Arch Ophthalmol 96:1653. 1978.

Streeten BW, Gibson SA, Li Z-Y: Lectin binding to pseudoexfoliative material and the ocular zonules. Invest Ophthalmol Vis Sci 27:1516, 1986.

RETINA 11

The retina is a highly specialized nervous tissue, in reality a part of the brain that has become exteriorized. It has the equivalent of both white matter (retinal plexiform and nerve fiber layers) and gray matter (retinal nuclear and ganglion cell layers). The glial cells are represented mostly by the very large, all pervasive, special Müller cells and, less noticeably, by the smaller astrocytes (and possible oligodendrocytes) of the inner retinal layers. As in the brain, a vasculature is present in which the endothelial cells possess tight junctions, producing a blood–retinal barrier. The retina, therefore, is susceptible to many diseases of the central nervous system, as well as to those diseases affecting tissues in general. Additionally, the highly specialized photoreceptor cells are subject to their own particular disorders.

Numerous congenital anomalies may involve the retina. These range from common disorders, such as albinism, to rare disorders, such as Oguchi's disease. Another common anomaly is the presence of myelinated nerve fibers; this generally occurs contiguous with the optic nerve head in the nerve fiber layer, but also may appear as an isolated retinal lesion. Lange's fold is routinely seen in histological sections of infant eyes, but it is a fixation artifact which is not present in vivo.

Vascular diseases often involve the retina. The retina is one of the few places in the body where blood vessels can be viewed directly. Signs of diseases such as diabetes mellitus (see Chapter 15) may therefore be viewed directly and detected in their early stages. Retinal ischemia is caused by anything that obstructs the passage of blood through the arteries and arterioles. Hemorrhagic retinopathy, on the other hand, is caused by an occlusion (partial or complete) of blood leaving the retina via the venules and veins. Arteriolarsclerosis and hypertension leave distinctive signs on the retinal arterioles. Clinical examination of the retina, therefore, may give some clues as to the status of lipid deposition and an indication of the level of the severity and chronicity of systemic blood pressure in the arterioles and arteries.

Symptoms of systemic diseases, such as sickle cell anemia and disseminated intravascular coagulation, can be detected in the retina, as can be unique entities such as Eales' disease and the retinopathy of prematurity (see Chapter 18).

Inflammations of all types may involve the retina. The pathology of such inflammations is similar to that of inflammations in general and has been covered in Chapters 3 and 4. Injuries have been discussed in Chapter 5.

Degenerations commonly involve the retina. Many degenerations (such as microcystoid and paving stone degeneration), although quite common, are of little or no clinical significance. Other degenerations (for example drusen) may lead to very serious abnormalities, like macular degeneration. Degenerations may occur: in highly myopic eyes; following ingestion of certain drugs, such as chloroquine (toxic retinopathy); or after radiotherapy near the eye (postradiation retinopathy). Degenerations may result from previous injuries or as a consequence of exposure to noxious agents of many different types.

Dystrophies, on the other hand, are primary afflictions of the retina. In general, dystrophies tend to be rare, to run in families, and to be bilaterally symmetrical. The pathology of many dystrophies has not been described. Some dystrophies, e.g., Stargardt's disease and fundus flavimaculatus, have only recently been characterized. The pathology of retinitis pigmentosa has been known for a long time, but its cause is unknown.

The retina may be involved secondarily in hereditary disease. Angioid streaks may be found in pseudoxanthoma elasticum, fibrodysplasia hyperelastica (Ehlers–Danlos syndrome), osteitis deformans (Paget's disease), sickle cell anemia, or may be idiopathic. The mucolipidoses (e.g., fucosidosis) mostly involve the anterior part of the eye, especially the cornea, but also may involve the retina. The sphingolipidoses (e.g., Tay–Sachs disease) often involve the retina, accentuating the normal fovea ("macular") cherry red spot.

Systemic diseases may affect the retina. The most common of these, diabetes mellitus, is discussed in Chapter 15. Tumors may arise from the retinal pigment epithelium (see Chapter 17), from the neurons (retinoblastoma, see Chapter 18), on a congenital basis (phakomatoses, see Chapter 2), or from the glial elements. The glial cells may proliferate, as noted in "cellophane maculopathy", where the cells grow out of the retina onto its internal surface and form an epiretinal membrane. Benign neoplasms may develop, such as a benign astrocytoma. Malignant glial neoplasms almost never occur. Very rarely metastases to the retina are found.

Retinal detachment, a separation of the neural retina from the retinal pigment epithelium, has many causes. In general, the detachment may be caused by: an abnormality of the choroid, causing fluid to collect under the retina; vitreous membranes which, through traction, pull the neural retina away from the pigment epithelium; or after a retinal tear (a rhegmatogenous retinal detachment). Following a retinal detachment due to any cause, the external (outer) layers of the retina are removed from their choriocapillaris blood supply and degenerate.

Fig. 11.1 CONGENITAL ANOMALIES OF THE RETINA

Albinism	Nonattachment
Grouped pigmentation	Retinal cysts
Coloboma	Myelination
Retinal dysplasia	Oguchi's disease
Lange's fold	Foveomacular anomalies

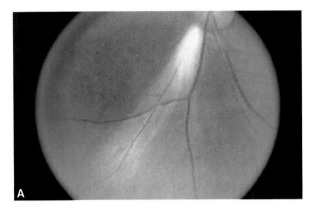

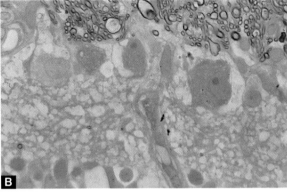

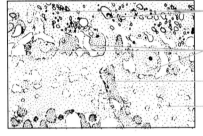

Fig. 11.2 Myelinated Nerve Fibers. A The myelinated nerve fibers fan out from the vicinity of the optic disc. The edges tend to be "feathered". **B** A histologic section shows that the nerve fiber layer, just anterior to (above) the ganglion cell layer, is thickened by heavy myelination. (**B**, PD.)

Myelination of nerve fiber layer axons

Ganglion cells

Capillary

Inner plexiform layer

Fig. 11.3 VASCULAR DISEASES OF THE RETINA

Retinal ischemia
Hemorrhagic infarction
Hypertensive retinopathy
Arteriolarsclerotic retinopathy
Diabetes mellitus (see Chapter 15)
Coats' (Leber's) disease (see Chapter 18)
Familial retinal telangiectasia

Retinal arteriolar macroaneurysms
Sickle cell disease
Eales' disease
Retinopathy of prematurity (see Chapter 18)
Hemangioma (capillary, cavernous)
Rendu–Osler–Weber disease (hereditary hemorrhagic telangiectasia)

Fig. 11.4 RETINAL ISCHEMIA HISTOLOGY

Early
Coagulative necrosis of inner retinal layers
Cotton wool spots

Late
Outer half of retina preserved
Inner half shows "homogenized scar"

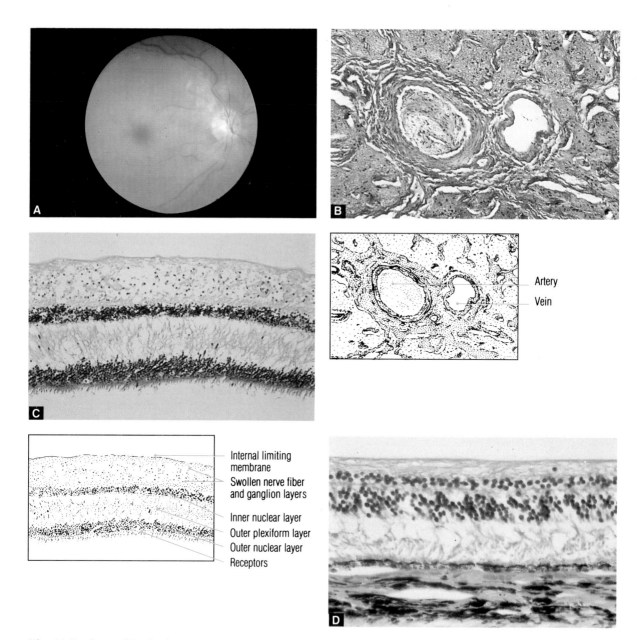

Fig. 11.5 Central Retinal Artery Occlusion. A The choriocapillaris shows through the central fovea (the thinnest area of the retina) as a red spot. The surrounding, thickened, edematous retina accentuates the normal red spot (which is also called a "cherry red spot"). The retinal arteries are attenuated. **B** The central retinal artery (on the left within the optic nerve), contains an organized thrombus. **C** The early stage of retinal ischemia shows edema of the inner retinal layers and pyknosis of ganglion cell nuclei. **D** The late stage of retinal occlusion (after healing) shows a homogeneous, diffuse, acellular scar replacing the inner plexiform, ganglion cell, and nerve fiber layers. (**A,** from *Ocular Pathology*, 2nd edn, by M Yanoff and BS Fine; **B**, trichrome.)

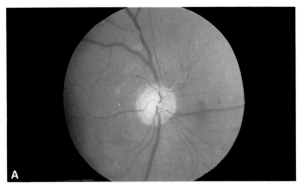

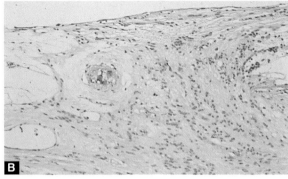

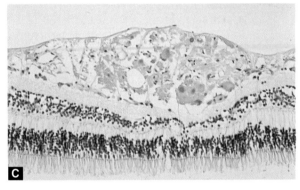

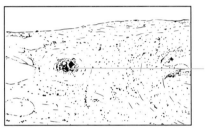

Cholesterol emboli in retinal artery

Fig. 11.6   Emboli. A A cholesterol embolus is seen in a tiny vessel just temporal to the optic disc. Scattered cotton wool spots also are present. **B** A histologic section of the same eye shows an intraarterial embolus composed of cholesterol crystals, surrounded by foreign body giant cells. **C** A histologic section of a cotton wool spot from another case shows a microinfarct of the nerve fiber layer. The individual nerve fibers are swollen and seen as round, pink areas, each of which contains a central dark spot (the altered swollen end bulb of the axon). These structures resemble cells and hence are called cytoid bodies.

Fig. 11.7 RETINAL VEIN OCCLUSION

Central retinal vein occlusion

Primary open-angle glaucoma is present in 8–20% of cases

Rubeosis iridis is seen in 55–65% of cases within the first 6 weeks to 6 months after an ischemic type of occlusion of the central retinal vein

Branch retinal vein occlusion

Neovascularization of the disc or retina may develop, especially if extensive capillary nonperfusion (ischemia) is present in the area of the occlusion

Histology

Early

Hemorrhage is present throughout the retinal layers

The normal retinal architecture is disrupted

Late

Healing occurs by proliferation of glial cells and further disruption of the architectural pattern

Special histologic stains indicate that iron is distributed widely throughout the retina (hemosiderosis)

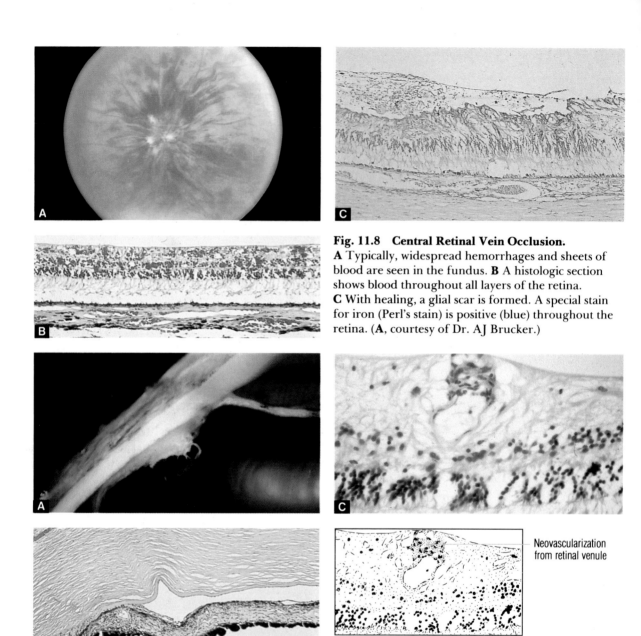

Fig. 11.8 Central Retinal Vein Occlusion.
A Typically, widespread hemorrhages and sheets of
blood are seen in the fundus. **B** A histologic section
shows blood throughout all layers of the retina.
C With healing, a glial scar is formed. A special stain
for iron (Perl's stain) is positive (blue) throughout the
retina. (**A**, courtesy of Dr. AJ Brucker.)

Neovascularization
from retinal venule

**Fig. 11.9 Complications of Central Retinal Vein
Occlusion. A** A gross specimen shows
neovascularization of the iris that has resulted in a
peripheral anterior synechia. **B** A histologic section
shows tissue present anterior to the anterior border
layer of the iris and between the peripheral iris and
the cornea. The tissue is neovascular (fibrous tissue
and blood vessels) tissue. **C** New blood vessels are
shown budding off from a retinal vein in this example
of early retinal neovascularization.

Fig. 11.10 OCULAR FINDINGS IN SICKLE CELL ANEMIA

Peripheral vessel disease, especially
  occlusion of arterioles

Peripheral whitening of retina

Retinitis proliferans ("sea fans")

Vitreous hemorrhage

Retinal detachment

Preretinal hemorrhages
  ("salmon patches")

Pigmented chorioretinal lesions
  ("black sunburst sign")

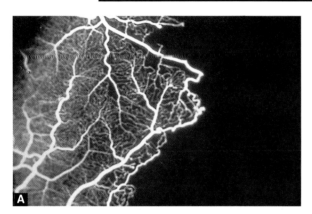

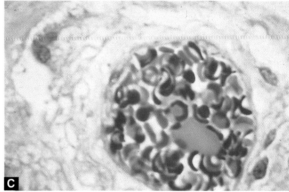

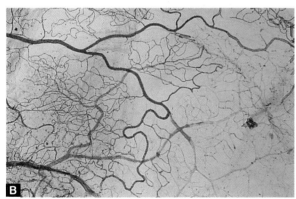

Fig. 11.11 Sickle Cell Hemoglobin C Disease.
A The perfusion of the retina stops abruptly at the equator, resulting in nonperfusion of the peripheral retina. **B** Trypsin digestion of the equatorial region of the retina (in this case, of sickle cell hemoglobin C disease) shows that peripheral blood vessels are devoid of cells and are nonviable. Arteriolar–venular collaterals are noted in the equatorial region. **C** A peripheral arteriole is occluded by sickled red blood cells. (**B**, PAS; **C**, MB, case shown here reported by Eagle RC, et al.: Arch Ophthalmol 92:28, 1974.)

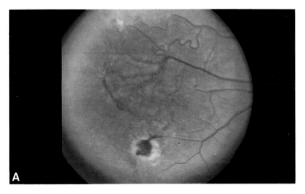

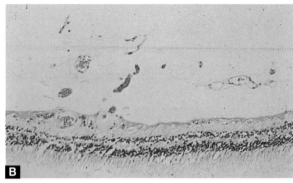

Fig. 11.12 Sickle Cell Hemoglobin C Disease.
A A sea fan is present at the equator and a sunburst is seen below the sea fan. **B** A histologic section shows that the sea fan lies between the internal surface of the retina and the vitreous body. The neovascularization is seen to proceed from a retinal arteriole into the subvitreal space and then back into a retinal venule. (**A**, courtesy of Dr. MF Rabb.)

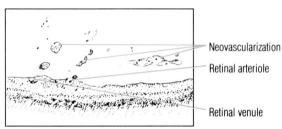

Neovascularization

Retinal arteriole

Retinal venule

Fig. 11.13 DEGENERATIONS

Microcystoid	Drusen	Toxic
Primary retinoschisis	Albinotic spots	Postirradiation
Secondary retinoschisis	Myopic	Traumatic
Paving stone	Macular	

Fig. 11.14 TYPICAL MICROCYSTOID DEGENERATION AND RETINOSCHISIS

Typical microcystoid degeneration	**Typical (senile adult) retinoschisis**
Consists of an intraretinal space less than one disc diameter in size	Consists of an intraretinal space greater than one disc diameter in size
A universal finding	Present in 4% of patients and is bilateral in 80%
	Rare under 20 years of age
Bilateral, superior temporal	Inferior temporal, 70%; superior temporal, 25%
	Small holes in the inner wall, larger outer-wall holes
Starts at ora serrata and extends posteriorly and circumferentially	Tends not to progress posteriorly
Contains hyaluronic acid within intraretinal spaces	Contains hyaluronic acid within intraretinal spaces
The pathology involves the middle retinal layers	The pathology involves the middle retinal layers

Fig. 11.15 RETICULAR MICROCYSTOID DEGENERATION AND RETINOSCHISIS

Reticular microcystoid degeneration

Present in 13% of autopsy eyes and in every decade of life

Bilateral in 41%

Inferior and superior temporal areas involved

It starts posterior to typical microcystoid degeneration

Contains hyaluronic acid within intraretinal spaces

The pathology involves the inner retinal layers (quite similar to that seen in juvenile retinoschisis)

Reticular retinoschisis

Present in 2% of autopsies and is rare under 30 years of age

Bilateral in 16%

Inferior temporal quadrant most common

Round or oval holes in the inner layer; rare outer-layer holes

The pathology involves the inner retinal layers (quite similar to that seen in juvenile retinoschisis)

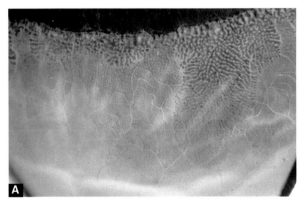

Fig. 11.16 Typical and Reticular Microcystoid Degeneration. A Typical microcystoid degeneration is seen to start just posterior to the ora serrata. Reticular cystoid degeneration is present just posterior to the typical microcystoid degeneration. **B** A transitional zone from typical (middle retinal layers) to reticular (inner retinal layers) cystoid degeneration is seen. The typical microcystoid degeneration is to the right (shown under increased magnification in **C**). (**B** and **C**, courtesy of Dr. RY Foos.)

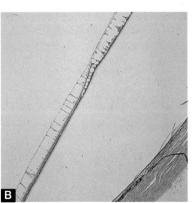

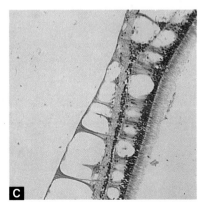

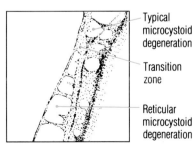

Typical microcystoid degeneration

Transition zone

Reticular microcystoid degeneration

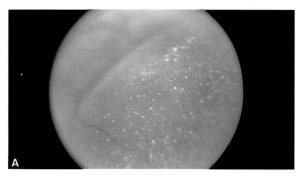

Fig. 11.17 Typical and Reticular Retinoschisis.
A A large, dome-shaped retinoschisis is present. Glistening, yellow-white dots are seen on its surface. **B** A histologic section shows typical retinoschisis. In order to determine whether retinoschisis is typical or reticular, the beginning part of the lesion (to the left) needs to be examined. Here the lesion is noted to start in the middle retinal layers. **C** A histologic section of reticular retinoschisis shows that the lesion starts in the inner retinal layers.

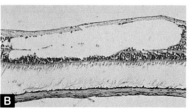

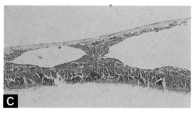

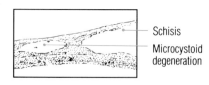

Schisis

Microcystoid degeneration

Fig. 11.18 PAVING STONE DEGENERATION

Incidence: 22–40% of patients	It does not make the eye more susceptible to retinal detachment
Inferior and temporal quadrants	Degeneration of outermost retinal layers and RPE

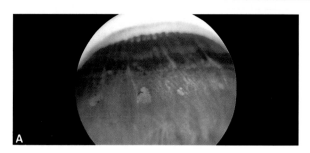

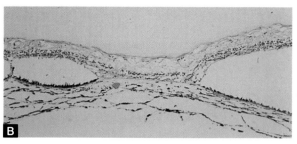

Fig. 11.19 Paving Stone Degeneration.
A Examination of the gross specimen shows nonelevated, sharply demarcated, yellow-white lesions which are present between the ora serrata and the equator. These lesions may extend and become confluent. **B** The retinal pigment epithelium ends abruptly in the area of degeneration. Bruch's membrane remains intact, but the overlying retina and the underlying choroid are atrophic.

Fig. 11.20 IDIOPATHIC MACULAR DEGENERATION

Precursors	Types
Central serous chorioretinopathy	"Dry" (atrophic)—no subretinal neovascularization(SRN)
Detachment of the retinal pigment epithelium	"Wet" (exudative, disciform)—SRN present
Drusen maculopathy	

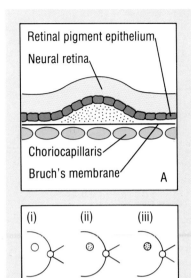
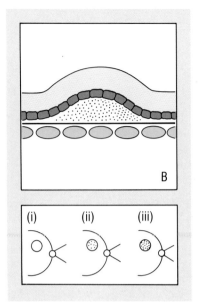
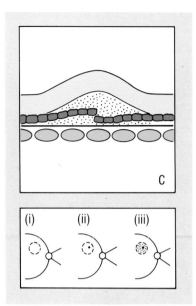

Fig. 11.21   Detachments of the Retinal Pigment Epithelium and Neural Retina. The schematic histology drawings in the upper panels correspond with the schematic drawings of the fundus pictures in the lower panels. **A** A simple, small retinal pigment epithelium (RPE) detachment. **B** A large RPE detachment. **C** A small RPE detachment with an overlying neural retina (NR) serous detachment. The triple drawings of the fundus represent (i) before fluorescein injection, (ii) the early fluorescein stage, and (iii) the late fluorescein stage. Note that the RPE detachments are sharply demarcated and fill completely with fluorescein in the late stage, whereas the NR serous detachment has fuzzy borders and does not fill completely with fluorescein in the late stage. (Adapted from Fig. 11–39 in *Ocular Pathology*, 2nd edn, by M Yanoff and BS Fine.)

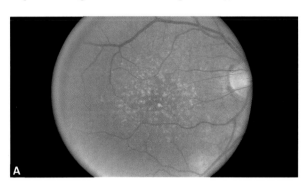
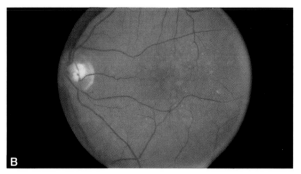

Fig. 11.22   Drusen. A The fundus picture shows small, "hard" drusen. Hard drusen appear to predipose the eye to the development of geographic atrophy of the RPE ("dry" macular degeneration). **B** Large, "soft" drusen are present. Soft drusen appear to result from the production of large amounts of abnormal basement membrane material which accumulates between the RPE and Bruch's membrane. The soft drusen seem to predispose the eye to subretinal neovascularization ("wet" macular degeneration). (**A**, courtesy of Dr. RC Eagle, Jr.)

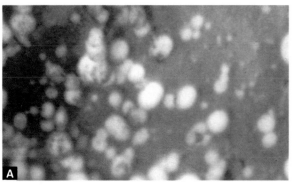

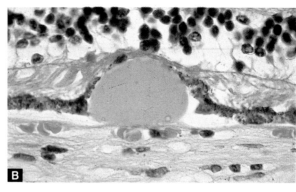

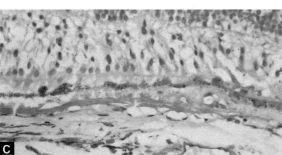

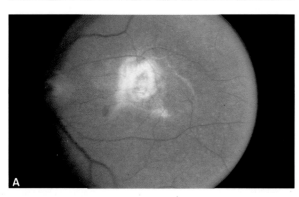

Fig. 11.23 Drusen. A In this gross specimen, the neural retina has been removed. The drusen are seen to protrude from the choroid and RPE. **B** A hard druse appears as a collection of basement membrane material between the attenuated RPE and Bruch's membrane. **C** In this example, confluent drusen are present, analagous to the soft drusen seen clinically. Small blood vessels are present within the drusen.

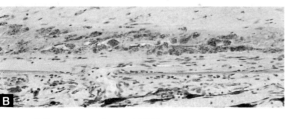

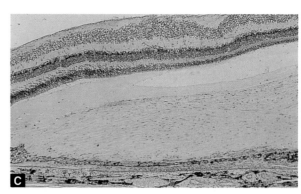

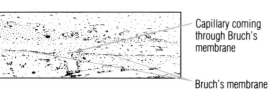

Capillary coming through Bruch's membrane

Bruch's membrane

Fig. 11.24 Disciform (Wet) Macular Degeneration. A The patient had subretinal neovascularization followed by numerous episodes of hemorrhage, resulting in an organized scar. **B** A small vessel has grown through Bruch's membrane into the subRPE space, resulting in hemorrhage and fibroplasia. **C** The end stage of the process shows a thick, fibrous scar between the choroid and outer retinal layers. Note the good preservation of the retina, except for the complete degeneration of the receptors. (Case shown in **B** reported in Frayer WC, Arch Ophthalmol 53:82, 1955.)

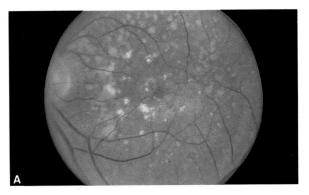

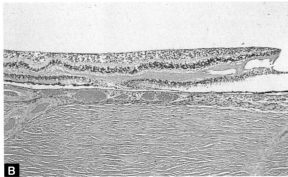

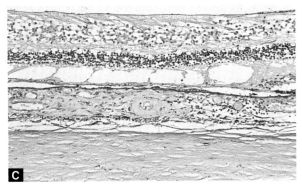

Retina
Bruch's membrane
Choroid
Thrombosed choroidal artery
Sclera

Fig. 11.25 Atrophic (Dry) Macular Degeneration.
A The patient showed drusen and abnormalities of the RPE in the form of increased translucency and pigment mottling, along with pigment loss. No subretinal neovascularization (SRN) was present in this eye. However, SRN was present in the fellow eye. **B** A histologic section of another eye shows irregular degeneration of the RPE, the outer retinal layers, and cystic changes in the outer plexiform layer. **C** A histologic section at another level of the same eye shows similar retinal changes along with a thrombus in a choroidal artery. Whether the choroidal thrombosis is related to the retinal changes in atrophic macular degeneration is not known. (**C**, from *Ocular Pathology*, 2nd edn, by M Yanoff and BS Fine.)

Fig. 11.26 HEREDITARY PRIMARY RETINAL DYSTROPHIES

Juvenile retinoschisis
Choroidal (choriocapillaris, gyrate, central areolar, serpiginous)
Stargardt's disease and fundus flavimaculatus
Retinitis pigmentosa (RP), peripheral and central
Retinitis punctata albescens (may be a form of RP)
Dominant drusen
Dominant cystoid macular dystrophy
Fenestrated sheen macular dystrophy

Vitelliform (Best's)
Dominant progressive foveal dystrophy
Progressive cone dystrophy
Crystalline retinopathy
Macular pattern (reticular, spider, butterfly)
Pseudoinflammatory dystrophy
Pigment epithelial dystrophy
Central areolar pigment epithelial dystrophy

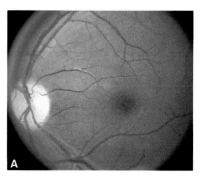

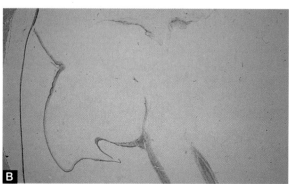

Fig. 11.27 Juvenile Retinoschisis. A The characteristic foveal lesion, resembling a polycystic fovea, is seen. Typically, no leakage is present when fluorescein angiography is performed. **B** A histologic section of another eye shows a large, temporal, peripheral retinoschisis cavity. **C** A histologic section of another area of the same eye shows a splitting in the ganglion and nerve fiber layers of the retina, the earliest finding in juvenile retinoschisis. The area of pathology is the same as that seen in reticular microcystoid degeneration and retinoschisis. (**A**, courtesy of Dr. AJ Brucker; case shown in **B** and **C** reported by Yanoff M, et al: Arch Ophthalmol 79:49, 1968.)

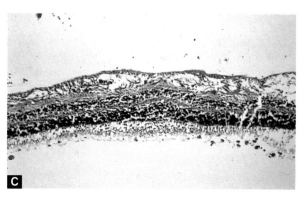

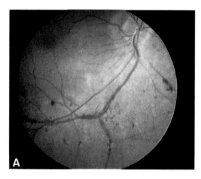

Fig. 11.28 Retinitis Pigmentosa. A The fundus picture shows a characteristic sharp demarcation from the relatively normal posterior pole to the "moth-eaten" appearance of the retina that extends out to the equator. Bone-corpuscular-shaped retinal pigmentation is present. **B** A histologic section of another case shows melanin-filled macrophages and RPE cells within the neural retina, mainly around blood vessels, resulting in the clinically seen bone-corpuscular-shaped pigmentation. **C** A histologic section of the posterior pole shows loss of receptors and atrophy of the choriocapillaris.

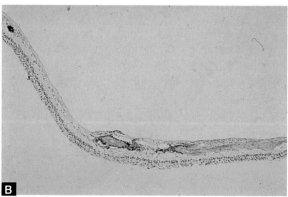

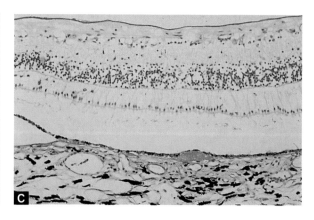

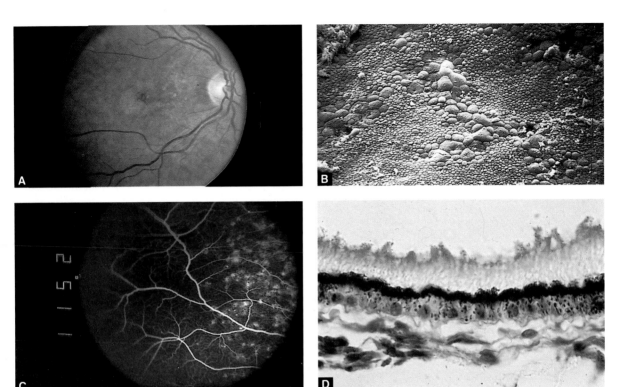

Fig. 11.29 Stargardt's Disease (Fundus Flavimaculatus). A Characteristic yellow-white flecks and an annular zone of foveal retinal pigment epithelial atrophy are present. **B** A scanning electron micrograph of an enucleated eye from the brother of the woman whose eye is shown in **A** demonstrates that the yellow-white flecks are caused by irregular, pisciform aggregates of enormous RPE cells, surrounded by a mosaic of smaller, relatively normal RPE cells. **C** Fluorescein angiography performed on the patient shown in **A** reveals a damping out of the background choroidal fluorescence (dark fundus), which is characteristic. **D** A histologic section, of the eye of the patient shown in **B**, shows that the fluorescein effect is caused by enlarged, lipofuscin-containing, RPE cells which act as a fluorescence filter. (Case shown in **B** and **D** reported by Eagle RC Jr, et al: Ophthalmology 7:1189, 1980.)

Fig. 11.30 HEREDITARY SECONDARY RETINAL DYSTROPHIES

Angioid streaks	Other lipidoses
Sjögren–Larsson syndrome	Disorders of carbohydrate metabolism
Mucopolysaccharidoses	Osteopetrosis
Mucolipidoses	Homocystinuria
Sphingolipidoses	

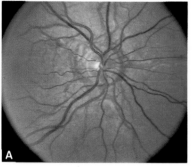
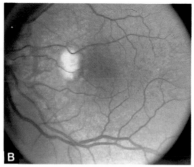
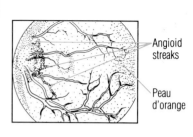

Angioid streaks

Peau d'orange

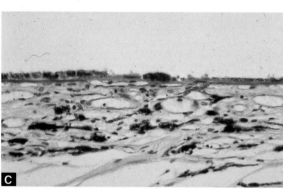

Fig. 11.31 Angioid Streaks. A A patient with angioid streaks also had pseudoxanthoma elasticum. The breaks in Bruch's membrane around the optic nerve resulted in angioid streaks. **B** Similar breaks away from the optic nerve have resulted in a "peau d'orange" appearance. The yellow area just temporal to the optic nerve represents subretinal neovascularization. **C** A histologic section of another case, from a patient with Paget's disease, shows that the streaks are caused by an interruption (break) in Bruch's membrane.

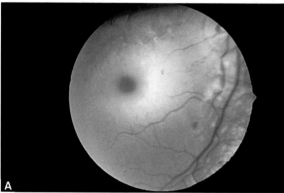

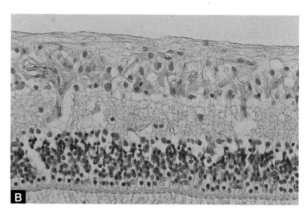

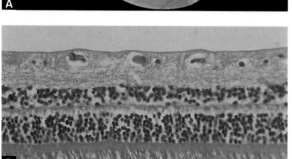

Fig. 11.32 Tay–Sachs Disease. A A characteristic cherry red spot is present in the central macula. **B** A histologic section shows a macular retina with a normal appearance, except for the ganglion cells which are swollen by PAS-positive material (sphingolipid). **C** The peripheral retina also shows ganglion cells where the cytoplasm is swollen by PAS-positive material. (**B, C**, PAS stain.)

Hereditary secondary retinal dystrophies
Diabetes mellitus (see Chapter 15)
Hypertension and arteriolarsclerosis
Collagen diseases
Blood dyscrasias
Demyelinating diseases (see Chapter 13)

Fig. 11.34 TUMORS OF THE RETINA

Glial (usual glial scar and massive gliosis)
Phakomatoses (see Chapter 2)
Retinal pigment epithelium (see Chapter 17)
Retinoblastoma (see Chapter 18)
Pseudogliomas (see Chapter 18)

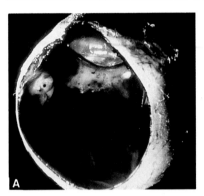

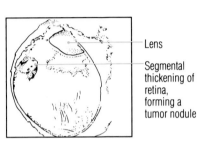

Lens

Segmental thickening of retina, forming a tumor nodule

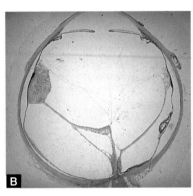

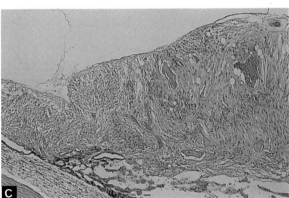

Fig. 11.35 **Massive Gliosis. A** Segmental thickening of the retina is seen in this gross specimen. The lesion was mistaken for a malignant melanoma and the eye was enucleated. **B** A histologic section of another case shows a sudden transition peripherally from a normal retinal thickness to a thickened, abnormal retina. **C** Massive gliosis is characterized histologically by total replacement and thickening of the retina by glial tissue and abnormal blood vessels. Frequently calcium and even inflammatory round cells are present within the tumor. (Cases shown in **A**, **B**, and **C** reported by Yanoff M, et al: Int Ophthalmol Clin 11:211, 1971.)

Fig. 11.36 MAJOR CAUSES OF RETINAL DETACHMENT

Fluid under intact sensory retina	**Traction bands in vitreous**
Harada's disease	Posttraumatic
Coats' disease	Diabetes
Malignant hypertension	**Fluid under broken sensory retina**
Eclampsia of pregnancy	Rhegmatogenous retinal detachment

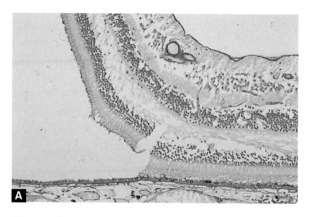

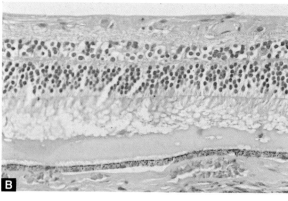

Fig. 11.37 Retinal Detachment. A An artifactitious retinal detachment (RD) shows no fluid in the subneural retinal space, pigment adherent to the tips of the photoreceptors, and good preservation of the normal retinal architecture in all layers. **B** A true RD shows material in the subneural retinal space and degeneration of the outer retinal layers.

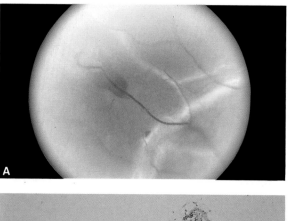

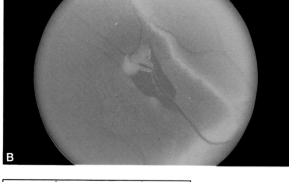

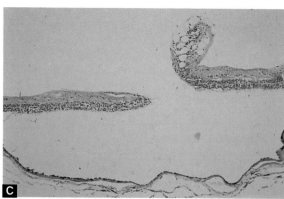

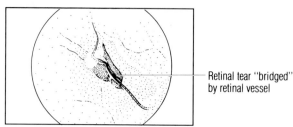

Retinal tear "bridged" by retinal vessel

Fig. 11.38 Horseshoe Retinal Tear. A The horseshoe retinal tear is not as easily seen with ordinary light as it is with red-free (green) light (**B**). **C** A histologic section shows the characteristic adherence of the vitreous to the anterior lip of the retinal tear and nonadherent to the posterior lip of the tear. (**B**, from *Ocular Pathology*, 2nd edn, by M Yanoff and BS Fine.)

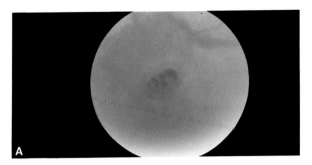

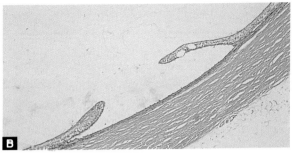

Fig. 11.39 Round Retinal Tear. A A round retinal
tear is surrounded by a small RD in the inferior retina.
B A histologic section shows that, in a round retinal
tear, vitreous is not adherent to the edge of the tear.
Note the rounded, smooth edges of the tear. An
artifactitious retinal tear has sharp edges. (**B**, courtesy
of Dr. WR Green.)

Fig. 11.40 PREDISPOSING FACTORS TO RETINAL DETACHMENT

Juvenile and senile retinoschisis
Lattice retinal degeneration
Cause of RD in 20–30% of patients with retinal detachment
Fewer than 1% of retinas with lattice acquire a detached retina

Retinal pits
Vitreoretinal adhesions
Trauma (surgical and nonsurgical)
Myopia
Diabetes mellitus

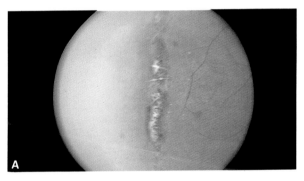

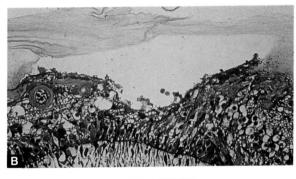

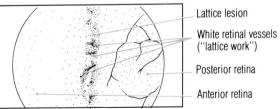

Lattice lesion
White retinal vessels
("lattice work")
Posterior retina
Anterior retina

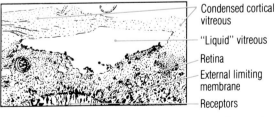

Condensed cortical
vitreous
"Liquid" vitreous
Retina
External limiting
membrane
Receptors

Fig. 11.41 Lattice Retinal Degeneration. A Heavy
pigmentation and thinning of the retina are present
circumferentially in an oval area. **B** The internal layers
of the retina, including the internal limiting
membrane, are not present. The overlying formed
vitreous is split (vitreoschisis) or separated from the
retina by fluid.

Fig. 11.42 PATHOLOGIC CHANGES FOLLOWING RETINAL DETACHMENT

Retinal atrophy	Demarcation lines
Subsensory retinal collections	Ringschwiele
Glial or RPE membrane growth	**Intraretinal cysts**
Fixed folds	**Calcium oxalate crystals**

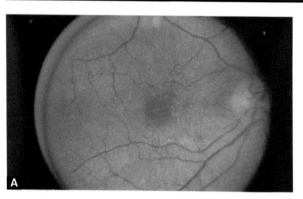

Fig. 11.43 Epiretinal (Flat) Gliosis. A The fundus shows characteristic crinkling or "cellophane appearance" of the retina in the posterior pole. **B** A histologic section of another case shows a fine, glial membrane on the internal surface of the retina. **C** A histologic section of a more advanced case shows that contraction of the glial membrane produced many folds of the internal surface of the retina.

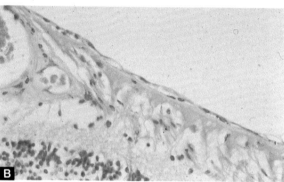

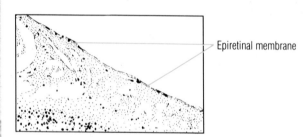

Epiretinal membrane

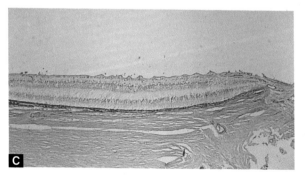

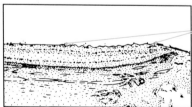

Wrinkled internal surface of the retina

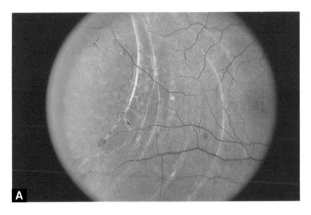

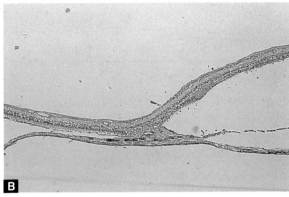

Fig. 11.44 Demarcation Line. A Concentric yellow-white lines are present at the edge of a RD. Some pigment also is present. **B** A histologic section shows the region of transition between retinal detachment and attachment. The RPE has undergone proliferation and the thickness of the basement membrane has increased. The yellow-white appearance of demarcation lines presumably is due to the basement membrane material. When the RPE cells are sufficiently pigmented, the demarcation lines will be pigmented. (**B**, courtesy Dr. WR Green.)

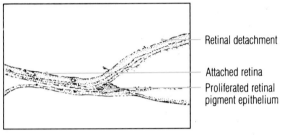

Retinal detachment

Attached retina

Proliferated retinal
pigment epithelium

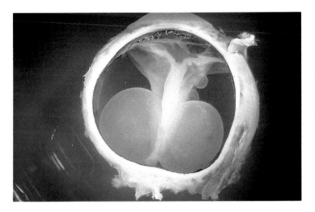

Fig. 11.45 Retinal Cysts. A This gross specimen shows numerous, large retinal cysts in this case of long-standing RD.

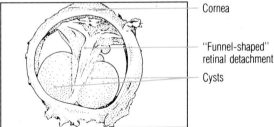

Cornea

"Funnel-shaped"
retinal detachment

Cysts

Bibliography

Aaby AA, Kushner BJ: Acquired and progressive myelinated nerve fibers. Arch Ophthalmol 103: 542, 1985.

Byer NE: The natural history of asymptomatic retinal breaks. Ophthalmology 89:1033, 1982.

Eagle RC, Jr: Mechanisms of maculopathy. Ophthalmology 91:613, 1984.

Eagle RC, Jr, et al: Retinal pigment epithelial abnormalities in fundus flavimaculatus. A light and electron microscopic study. Ophthalmology 7:1189, 1980.

Eagle RC, Jr, Yanoff M, Fine BS: Hemoglobin SC retinopathy and fat emboli to the eye. A light and electron microscopical study. Arch Ophthalmol 92:28, 1974.

Foos RY, Feman SS: Reticular cystoid degeneration of the peripheral retina. Am J Ophthalmol 69:392, 1970.

Foos RY, Simons KB: Vitreous in lattice degeneration of the retina. Ophthalmology 91:452, 1984.

Frangieh GT, et al: Histopathologic study of nine branch retinal vein occlusions. Arch Ophthalmol 100:1132, 1982.

Frayer WC: Elevated lesions of the macular area. A histopathologic study emphasizing lesions similar to disciform degeneration of the macula. Arch Ophthalmol 53:82, 1955.

Green WR, McDonnell PJ, Yeo JH: Pathologic features of senile macular degeneration. Ophthalmology 92:615, 1985.

Kampik A, et al: Epiretinal and vitreous membranes. Comparative study of 56 cases. Arch Ophthalmol 99:1445, 1981.

Magargal LE, Donoso LA, Sanborn GE: Retinal ischemia and risk of neovascularization following central retinal vein obstruction. Ophthalmology 89:1241, 1982.

McLane NJ, et al: Angioid streaks associated with hereditary spherocytosis. Am J Ophthalmol 97:444, 1984.

Miller H, Miller B, Ryan SJ: Newly formed subretinal vessels. Fine structure and fluorescein leakage. Invest Ophthalmol Vis Sci 27:204, 1986.

Patz A: Clinical and experimental studies on retinal neovascularization. XXXIX Edward Jackson Memorial Lecture. Am J Ophthalmol 94:715, 1982.

Pruett RC: Retinitis pigmentosa. Clinical observations and correlations. Trans Am Ophthalmol Soc 81:693, 1983.

Sarks SH: Drusen and their relationship to senile macular degeneration. Aust N Z J Ophthalmol 8:117, 1980.

Tso MOM: Pathogenetic factors of aging macular degeneration. Ophthalmology 92:628, 1985.

Yanoff M, Rahn EK, Zimmerman LE: Histopathology of juvenile retinoschisis. Arch Ophthalmol 79:49, 1968.

Yanoff M, Zimmerman LE, Davis R: Massive gliosis of the retina. A continuous spectrum of glial proliferation. Int Ophthalmol Clin 11:211, 1971.

VITREOUS 12

The vitreous body is one of the most delicate and transparent of connective tissues. It occupies the posterior or larger compartment of the eye, filling the globe between the retina and the lens. The structure is composed of a framework of extremely delicate or embryonic collagen filaments closely associated with a large quantity of water binding hyaluronic acid.

Embryologically, the developing avascular secondary vitreous surrounds and compresses the vascularized primary vitreous into a canal. This canal (called the hyaloid canal, or the canal of Cloquet) contains the hyaloid vessel and extends from the optic disc to the back of the lens. With maturation, the hyaloid vessel atrophies to disappear before birth. Persistence of remnants of the primary vitreous produces congenital anomalies, the most common of which are retention of fragments on the back of the lens (Mittendorf dot), retention of tissue on the optic disc (Bergmeister's papilla), and persistent hyperplastic primary vitreous (see Chapter 18), which often encroaches on the tissue of the posterior lens.

Inflammatory diseases may involve the vitreous primarily or secondarily. The inflammations are quite similar to those already discussed in Chapters 3 and 4.

Vitreous adhesions, membranes, and opacities may form secondary to a variety of causes. They may be congenital, follow trauma, follow inflammation, be secondary to systemic or familial diseases, or be idiopathic. Hemorrhage into the vitreous is a common cause of loss of vision. Most frequently, hemorrhage occurs in a diabetic patient and is secondary to the presence of abnormal, easily ruptured vessels (see Chapter 15). Vitreous hemorrhage also may be secondary to trauma, retinal tears, vitreoretinal separation, hypertensive or sickle cell retinopathy, Eales' disease, retinal vascularization from any cause, disciform degeneration of the macula, blood dyscrasias, uveitis, malignant melanoma, retinoblastoma, metastatic intraocular tumors, Terson's syndrome (subarachnoid hemorrhage plus vitreous hemorrhage), retinal angiomas, juvenile retinoschisis, and choroidal hemorrhage with extension. Hemorrhage into the vitreous compartment, between the vitreous body and the internal surface of the retina, generally resorbs rapidly (within a few weeks to a few months). Hemorrhage into the vitreous body may be spontaneously reabsorbed (but it usually takes a considerable amount of time, i.e., 3 months or more), or it may organize and form fibrous membranes. The membranes shrink and cause traction on the retina, which may produce a retinal detachment (see Chapter 11). Glaucoma, in the form of hemolytic glaucoma (see Chapter 16) may also be a complication of an intravitreal hemorrhage.

FIG. 12.1 CONGENITAL ANOMALIES

Persistent primary vitreous

Anterior remnants: lenticular portion of hyaloid; Mittendorf dot

Posterior remnants: vascular loops; Bergmeister's papilla; congenital cysts

Anterior persistent hyperplastic primary vitreous (see Chapter 18)

Posterior persistent hyperplastic primary vitreous

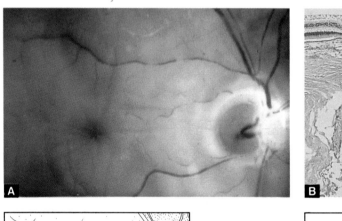

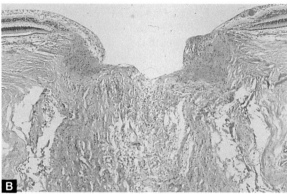

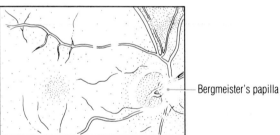

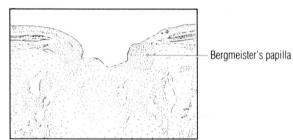

Fig. 12.2 Bergmeister's Papilla. A The enucleated eye shows posterior remnants of the hyaloid system over the nasal portion of the optic nerve head.

B histologic section shows a Bergmeister's papilla in the form of a glial remnant of the hyaloid system.

FIG. 12.3 VITREOUS

Inflammation (see Chapters 3 and 4)

Acute   Chronic

FIG. 12.4 POSTTRAUMATIC AND SURGICAL VITREOUS ADHESIONS

Vitreocorneal
Corneal "touch" syndrome
Iridovitreal
Posterior synechiae
Total synechiae lead to seclusion of pupil and iris bombé
Pupillary membrane leads to occlusion of pupil

Vitreoretinal
Irvine–Gass syndrome
"Cellophane" retina
Postinflammation
Idiopathic

FIG. 12.5 VITREOUS OPACITIES

Hyaloid vessel remnants
Acquired vitreous floaters
Posterior vitreous detachment
Present in more than 50% of patients over 50 years of age
Present in 65% of patients over 65 years of age
Proteinaceous deposits
Inflammatory cells
Red blood cells
Iridescent particles
Asteroid hyalosis—calcium soaps
Synchysis scintillans—cholesterol (see Fig. 5.24)
Tumor cells
Pigment dust
Cysts
Retinal fragments
Traumatic avulsion of vitreous base
Anterior vitreous detachment

Familial exudative vitreoretinopathy
Posterior vitreous detachment
Centrally organized vitreous membrane bound to the retina
Snowflake opacities
Retinal traction
Nonperfusion of the temporal retinal periphery and retinal neovascularization
Autosomal dominant
Amyloid
Primary familial
Sheet-like vitreous veils
Deposits in lids, orbit, nerves, and ganglia
Widespread systemic deposits
Histology shows pale, amorphous material that is Congo-red-positive, metachromatic, dichroic, and birefringent

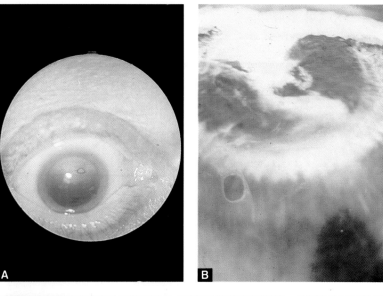

Fig. 12.6 Posterior Vitreous Detachment. A The fundus reflex shows the characteristic "donut" or "peep hole" of posterior vitreous detachment (PVD). **B** An enucleated eye shows the previous attachment site of the vitreous around the optic nerve, now floating freely in the central vitreous compartment as a round, fibrous band. **C** Another enucleated eye shows that the vitreous is detached posteriorly everywhere except around the optic nerve head. **D** The vitreous is detached posteriorly, except around the optic nerve head where it is attached to the edges of the nerve.

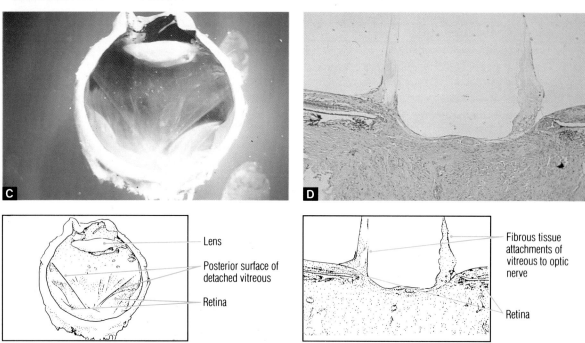

Lens

Posterior surface of detached vitreous

Retina

Fibrous tissue attachments of vitreous to optic nerve

Retina

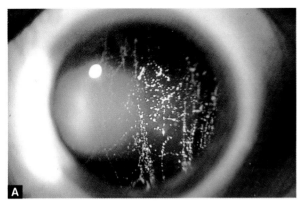

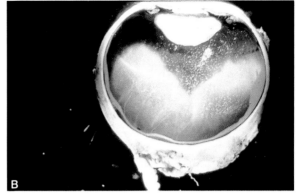

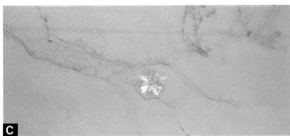

Fig. 12.7 Asteroid Hyalosis. A The fundus reflex shows tiny, gold-colored balls in the anterior vitreous. **B** The enucleated globe shows multiple, tiny, white spherules suspended throughout the vitreous body. **C** A histologic section shows that the tiny bodies are birefringent in polarized light.

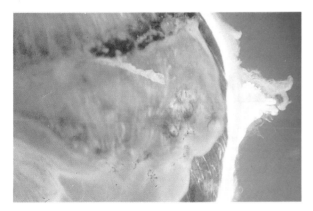

Ora serrata
Avulsed vitreous base
Traumatic chorioretinal atrophy
Retina

Fig. 12.8 Avulsion of the Vitreous Base. The vitreous base is seen to be partially avulsed. The patient had blunt injury to this eye.

FIG. 12.9 VITREOUS HEMORRHAGE

Definitions

Intravitreal—within the vitreous

Subvitreal—between the vitreous body and the internal surface of the retina

Subhyaloid—confusing term: a subhyaloid hemorrhage is usually actually within the retina, between the internal limiting membrane (ILM) and the nerve fiber layer of the retina (submembranous, intraretinal)

Causes

Retinal tears
Vitreoretinal separations
Trauma
Diabetic retinopathy
Hypertensive retinopathy
Sickle cell retinopathy
Eales' disease
Retinal neovascularization
Disciform macular degeneration
Choroidal hematoma
Juvenile retinoschisis
Blood dyscrasias
Uveitis
Malignant melanoma
Retinoblastoma
Metastatic tumor
Retinal angiomas
Subarachnoid hemorrhage (Terson's syndrome)

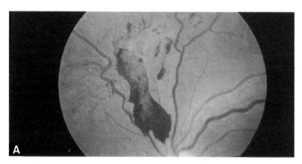

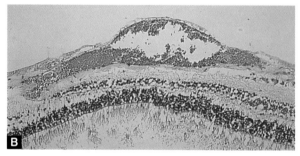

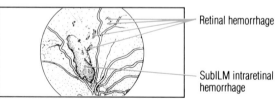

Retinal hemorrhage

SubILM intraretinal hemorrhage

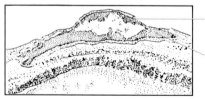

Internal surface of retina

SubILM intraretinal hemorrhage

Fig. 12.10 Submembranous Intraretinal Hemorrhage. A A hemorrhage is seen between the internal limiting membrane (ILM) and the nerve fiber layer of the retina. This is often mistakenly called a subhyaloid hemorrhage. **B** A histologic section of another case shows that the hemorrhage lies entirely within the retina, separated from the vitreous compartment by a thick basement membrane (ILM of the retina).

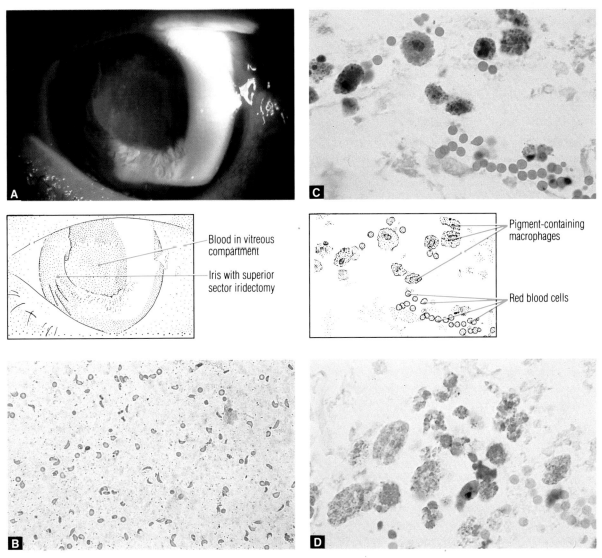

Blood in vitreous compartment

Iris with superior sector iridectomy

Pigment-containing macrophages

Red blood cells

Fig. 12.11 Intravitreal Hemorrhage. A A hemorrhage is seen within the vitreous body. **B** In this vitrectomy specimen of an intravitreal hemorrhage from a 67-year-old black man, the red blood cells were noted to have a sickle configuration; a diagnosis of sickle cell trait was made. The diagnosis had not been made previously. **C** Another vitrectomy specimen shows red blood cells and pigment-containing macrophages. **D** A special stain for iron (Perl's stain) shows that the pigment in some of the macrophages stains positively (blue), signifying hemosiderin; and pigment in other macrophages does not stain, and presumably represents melanin or hemoglobin not yet oxidized to hemosiderin. (**A**, courtesy of Dr. SH Sinclair.)

Bibliography

Boldrey EE, et al: The histopathology of familial exudative vitreoretinopathy. A report of two cases. Arch Ophthalmol 103:238, 1985.

Eagle RC, Jr, Yanoff M: Cholesterolosis of anterior chamber. Albrecht von Graefes Arch Klin Ophthalmol 193:121, 1975.

Foos RY: Posterior vitreous detachment. Trans Am Acad Ophthalmol Otolaryngol 76:480, 1972.

Forrester JV, Lee WR, Williamson J: The pathology of vitreous hemorrhage. I. Gross and histological appearances. Arch Ophthalmol 96:703, 1978.

Miller H, et al: Asteroid bodies—an ultrastructural study. Invest Ophthalmol Vis Sci 24:133, 1983.

Orellana J, et al: Pigmented free-floating vitreous cysts in two young adults. Electron microscopic observations. Ophthalmology 92:297, 1985.

OPTIC NERVE 13

The optic nerve is made up of a number of components. White matter, in the form of glial supporting elements and axons from the retinal ganglion cells, is the major constituent. All the meningeal sheaths (dura, arachnoid, and pia) are present, along with an intrinsic and extrinsic blood supply. The optic nerve is continuous at one end with the retina and at the other end with the brain, making it vulnerable to a variety of ocular and central nervous system diseases.

Numerous anatomic variations and congenital defects may involve the optic nerve. These range from complete absence of the optic nerve (aplasia) to minor abnormalities, such as differences in the size and shape of the optic nerve head. An optic pit may be seen within the optic nerve head, usually in the inferotemporal quadrant. The pit may be associated with a serous detachment of the central (macular) retina.

Swelling of the optic nerve, manifested as optic disc edema, may have a local cause within the eye, may be an extension of an intracranial disorder, or be part of a systemic abnormality (such as malignant hypertension). The optic nerve may become inflamed, which results in a condition called optic neuritis. The inflammation may be caused by a local phenomenon, such as uveitis, or be part of a generalized condition, such as multiple sclerosis. Atrophy of the optic nerve may result from many diverse conditions. Whatever the cause, however, the histologic findings in optic atrophy are similar and reflect a loss of parenchyma (myelinated neurites) and an increase in glial cell mass, but not sufficient to compensate for the parenchymal loss.

The optic nerve may give rise to primary tumors, as in juvenile pilocytic astrocytoma (glioma) and meningioma, or may be the site of secondary tumors, due for instance to invasion by retinoblastoma or to leukemic involvement. Tumors can cause secondary effects, e.g., optic disc edema or optic atrophy.

FIG. 13.1 CONGENITAL DEFECTS AND ANATOMIC VARIATIONS

Aplasia	Congenital crescent or conus
Hypoplasia	Congenital optic atrophy
Dysplasia	Coloboma
Anomalous shape of optic disc and optic cup	Optic pit
	Myopia

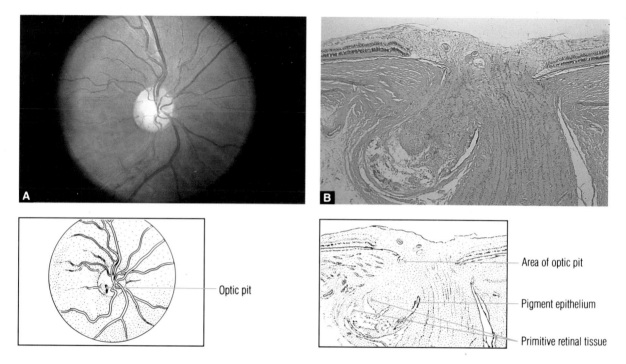

Fig. 13.2   Optic Pit. A A small, angular depression is present in the inferotemporal quadrant of the disc, which is the usual location for the pit. The patient had an associated detachment of the macular retina. **B** A histologic section of another case shows the herniation of retinal tissue through the enlarged scleral opening along one side of the optic nerve. An optic pit is a form of coloboma of the optic nerve. (**B**, courtesy of Dr. JB Crawford, reported in Irvine AR, et al: Retina 6:146, 1986.)

FIG. 13.3 OPTIC DISC EDEMA	
Causes	**Histology**
Increased venous pressure at or posterior to lamina cribrosa	Acute
Acute glaucoma	Edema, vascular congestion, increased volume of tissue, hemorrhages, and narrowing of physiologic cup
Brain tumors	
Increased venous pressure at or anterior to lamina cribrosa	Displacement of sensory retina away from the optic disc, and peripapillary retinal and choroidal folds
Ocular hypotony	
Central retinal vein occlusion	Peripapillary retinal detachment
Local phenomena	Chronic
Irvine–Gass syndrome	Degeneration of nerve fibers
Iron deficiency anemia	Gliosis and optic atrophy

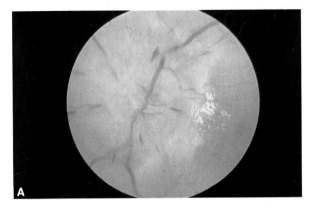

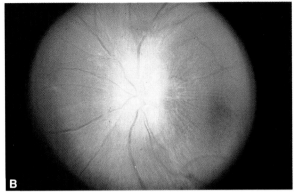

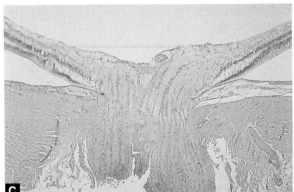

Fig. 13.4 Optic Disc Edema. A The acutely swollen optic nerve head is surrounded by concentric retinal folds. Note the retinal flame-shaped hemorrhages and exudates. The patient had severe hypertension. **B** This patient had chronic, bilateral optic disc edema, secondary to an orbital pseudotumor. **C** A histologic section of another case of acute optic disc edema shows the characteristic findings. Increased mass is caused by axonal swelling, tissue edema, and vascular congestion. The photoreceptors are displaced laterally from Bruch's membrane, which terminates in a ring at the optic nerve. (**C**, from *Ocular Pathology*, 2nd edn, by M Yanoff and BS Fine.)

FIG. 13.5 PSEUDOPAPILLEDEMA	**FIG. 13.6 CAUSES OF OPTIC NEURITIS** 
Hypermetropic optic disc Drusen of optic nerve head Congenital developmental abnormalities Optic neuritis and perineuritis Myelinated (medullated) nerve fibers	**Secondary to ocular disease** Keratitis Uveitis Endophthalmitis **Secondary to orbital disease** Cellulitis Thrombophlebitis Arteritis **Secondary to intracranial disease** Meningitis **Secondary to vascular disease** Temporal arteritis **Secondary to demyelinating disease** **Secondary to spread of distant infection** **Secondary to nutritional, toxic, or metabolic processes** Tobacco–alcohol amblyopia **Secondary to hereditary conditions** **Secondary to idiopathic causes**

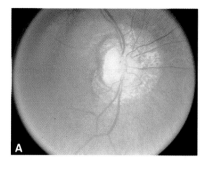

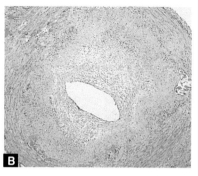

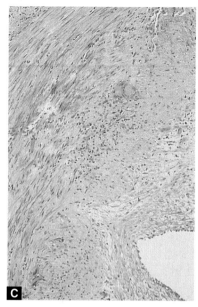

Fig. 13.7 Temporal Arteritis. A The patient had a gradual decrease in vision in his left eye along with generalized weakness and a 11.4 kg weight loss. The fundus shows an atrophic optic nerve head as a result of temporal arteritis. **B** A histologic section of the temporal artery from this case shows a granulomatous, giant cell reaction in the inflamed wall of the artery. The internal elastic lamina of the artery is fragmented. **C** Increased magnification shows the giant cells and granulomatous inflammation.

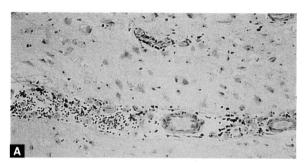

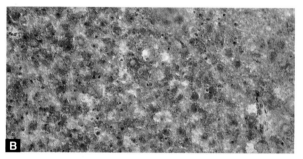

Fig. 13.8 Demyelinating Disease. A A histologic section of the occipital lobe from a patient who had Schilder's disease shows a marked perivascular inflammatory reaction, which consists mainly of lymphocytes and some plasma cells. The surrounding brain parenchyma demonstrates a reactive gliosis and contains a proliferation of astrocytes. **B** Special stains for fat (oil red-O) show considerable amounts of lipid present in the tissue.

FIG. 13.9 CAUSES OF OPTIC ATROPHY

Ascending Primary lesion in retina or optic disc (e.g., glaucoma), and secondary effects on the optic nerve and brain **Descending** Primary lesion in the optic nerve or brain (e.g., tabes dorsalis, hydrocephalus)	**Inherited** Leber's optic atrophy Behr's optic atrophy Friedreich's ataxia

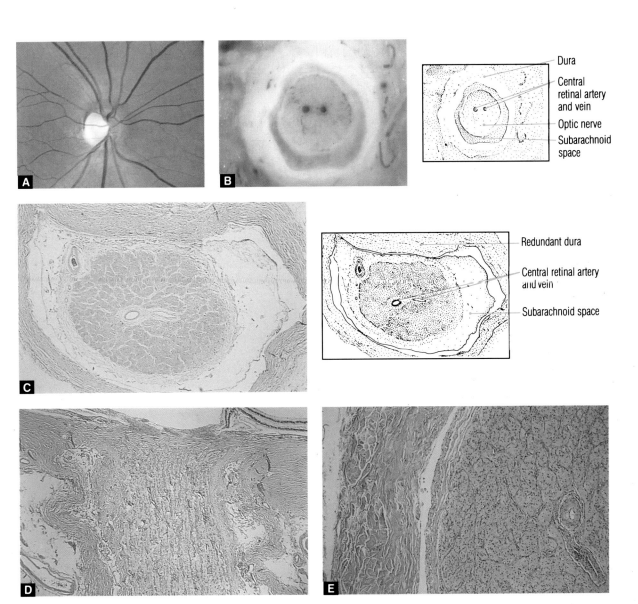

Fig. 13.10 Optic Atrophy. A The patient had
retrobulbar neuritis in this eye, leaving him with optic
atrophy of the temporal half of the optic nerve head.
B Gross examination of an enucleated eye in another
case shows marked atrophy of the parenchyma of the
optic nerve, which has resulted in a widened
subarachnoid space. **C** A histologic cross section shows
the optic nerve to be atrophic and shrunken, resulting
in an increased size of the subarachnoid space, a
redundancy of the dura, a widening of the pial septa,

and gliosis. **D** A longitudinal histologic section shows
that the optic nerve is of the same diameter where it
enters the eye as it is posterior to the sclera. Normally,
the optic nerve doubles in diameter behind the
sclera, because of the accumulation of myelin. The
narrowness of the optic nerve is due to atrophy.
The subarachnoid space is widened and the dura is
redundant. **E** Increased magnification of another case
shows the marked cellularity of the atrophic nerve
which is caused by proliferation of astrocytes.

FIG. 13.11 PRIMARY OPTIC NERVE TUMORS

Juvenile pilocytic astrocytoma ("glioma")	Medulloepithelioma
Oligodendrocytoma	Giant drusen (see Chapter 2)
Malignant astrocytoma	Ordinary drusen
Meningioma	Juxtapapillary retinal pigment epithelial drusen
Melanocytoma (see Chapter 17)	Corpora amylacea
Hemangioma	Corpora arenacea

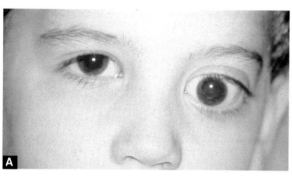

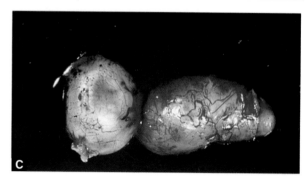

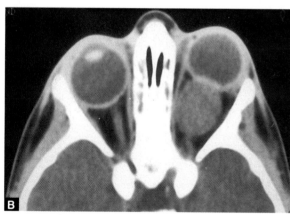

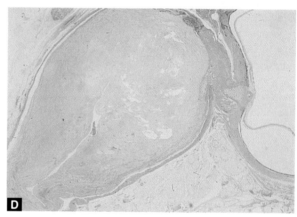

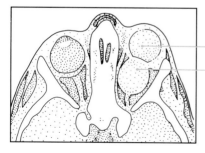

Proptotic eye

"Glioma" of optic nerve

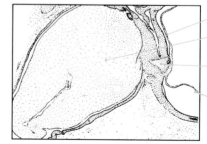

Sclera

Optic nerve glioma

Optic nerve

Retina

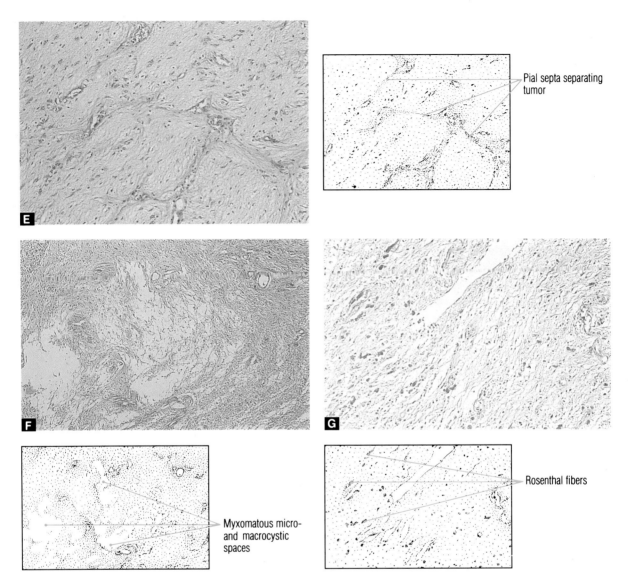

Fig. 13.12 Optic Nerve "Glioma". A The patient has
proptosis of the left eye caused by a glioma of the
optic nerve. Most of the time the proptosis is in a
down-and-out direction. B The CT scan of this case
shows the glioma enlarging the retrobulbar optic
nerve. C This gross specimen from another case shows
the optic nerve thickened by tumor, starting just
behind the globe. D A large tumor involves and
thickens the optic nerve. E Increased magnification
shows enlarged neural bundles between the spread
out pial septa. The neural bundles contain expanded,
disordered glial cells, and a few axons. F An area of
necrosis within the tumor shows myxomatous
microcystoid and macrocystoid spaces. G Many
astrocytes contain intracytoplasmic, eosinophilic
structures, called Rosenthal fibers. (A, B, case
presented by Dr. JA Shields at the Armed Forces
Institute of Pathology Alumni meeting, June 1987; C,
courtesy of Dr. WC Frayer; C, D, from *Ocular
Pathology*, 2nd edn, by M Yanoff and BS Fine.)

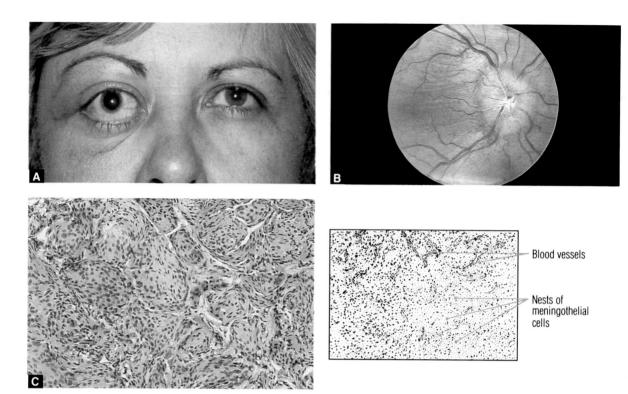

Fig. 13.13   Meningioma. A A meningioma of the orbital portion of the optic nerve has caused proptosis of the right eye. **B** Fundus examination shows optic disc edema of long-term duration. **C** A biopsy of another case shows a proliferation of meningothelial cells. As is often the case, no psammoma bodies are present. (**A, B,** courtesy of Dr. WC Frayer.)

Blood vessels

Nests of meningothelial cells

FIG. 13.14 SECONDARY OPTIC NERVE TUMORS

Retinoblastoma

Malignant melanoma

Hamartoma of retinal pigment epithelium

Metastatic carcinoma

Leukemia and lymphoma

Glioblastoma multiforme

Myelin artifact

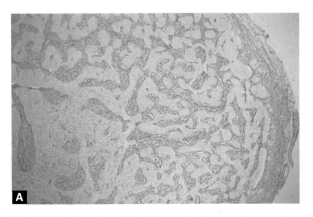

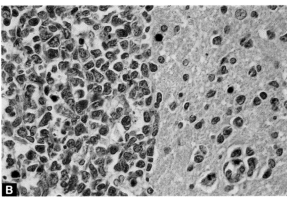

Fig. 13.15   Leukemic infiltrate. A The pial septa of the optic nerve are markedly thickened. The subarachnoid space contains a cellular infiltrate.

B Increased magnification shows that the pial septa are thickened by blastic leukemic cells.

Bibliography

Apple DJ, Rabb MF, Walsh PM: Congenital anomalies of the optic disc (Review). Surv Ophthalmol 27:3, 1982.

Arnold AC, et al: Retinal periphlebitis and retinitis in multiple sclerosis. I. Pathologic characteristics. Ophthalmology 91:255, 1984.

Borodic GE, et al: Peripapillary subretinal neovascularization and serous macular detachment. Association with congenital optic nerve pits. Arch Ophthalmol 102:229, 1984.

Hayreh SS: Fluids in the anterior part of the optic nerve in health and disease. Surv Ophthalmol 23:1, 1978.

Imes RK, et al: Evolution of optociliary veins in optic nerve sheath meningiomas. Arch Ophthalmol 103:59, 1985.

Irvine AR, Crawford JB, Sullivan JH: The pathogenesis of retinal detachment with morning glory disc and optic pit. Retina 6:146, 1986.

Kincaid MC, Green WR: Ocular and orbital involvement in leukemia (Review). Surv Ophthalmol 27:211, 1983.

Kivlin JD, et al: Linkage analysis in dominant optic atrophy. Am J Hum Genet 35:1190, 1983.

Quigley HA, Miller NR, Green WR: The pattern of optic nerve fiber loss in anterior ischemic optic neuropathy. Am J Ophthalmol 100:769, 1985.

Roth AM, Milsow L, Keltner JL: The ultimate diagnosis of patients undergoing temporal artery biopsies. Arch Ophthalmol 102:901, 1984.

Sher NA, et al: Unilateral papilledema in 'benign' intracranial hypertension (pseudotumor cerebri). JAMA 250:2346, 1983.

Sibony PA, et al: Optic nerve sheath meningiomas. Clinical manifestations. Ophthalmology 91:1313, 1984.

Yanoff M, Davis R, Zimmerman LE: Juvenile pilocytic astrocytoma ("glioma") of optic nerve: clinicopathologic study of 63 cases. In Jakobiec FA (ed): Ocular and Adexal Tumors, p. 685, Birmingham: Aesculapius Publishing Company, 1978.

ORBIT 14

In addition to the eye and the optic nerve, the orbit contains many soft tissue structures such as fat, muscle (striated and nonstriated), cartilage, bone, fibrous tissue, nerves, and blood vessels. Orbital disease, whatever its cause, tends to increase the bulk of the orbit, so the main presenting sign is exophthalmos. Other than the epithelia in the eye, the lacrimal gland is the only epithelial structure within the orbit. All orbital structures may be involved in disease processes. Many congenital anomalies may affect both the bony structure of the orbit as well as the soft tissues within the orbit. Inflammatory diseases of all types may affect the orbit. Inflammation has already been discussed in general in Chapters 3 and 4.

Many systemic diseases may involve the orbit. The most important of these is Graves' disease. Graves' disease is one of the most common causes of exophthalmos.

Orbital tumors may arise initially in the orbit, extend into the orbit from contiguous structures, or secondarily affect the orbit from distant sites (metastatic). Congenital tumors that contain tissue normally present (such as blood vessels) are called hamartomas. Congenital tumors that contain tissue not normally present (e.g., hair follicles) are called choristomas. Many mesenchymal tumors may arise from orbital soft tissues. The most important of these are fibrous histiocytoma and rhabdomyosarcoma. Numerous neural tumors involve the orbit. Neurofibroma has been described in Chapter 2. Glioma of the optic nerve and meningoma have been described in Chapter 13. Neurilemmoma is illustrated in this chapter (Fig. 14.18).

The major epithelial tumors found in the orbit arise from the lacrimal gland. The most common benign lacrimal gland tumor is the benign mixed tumor. The most common malignant tumor is adenoid cystic carcinoma. Lymphoid lesions, both benign and malignant, and leukemias often involve the orbit. In fact, lymphoid lesions and Graves' disease are the commonest causes of exophthalmos. Other diseases, such as fibrous dysplasia and Langerhans' granulomatoses (histiocytosis X) may effect the orbit. The most common entity involving the orbit in the group of Langerhans' granulomatoses is eosinophilic granuloma.

FIG. 14.1 DEVELOPMENTAL ABNORMALITIES

Developmental abnormalities of bony orbit
Microphthalmos with cyst
Cephaloceles
Congenital alacrima

FIG. 14.3 INJURIES (SEE CHAPTER 5)

Penetrating wounds
Nonpenetrating wounds

FIG. 14.4 VASCULAR DISEASE

Primary
Varix
Cavernous sinus thrombosis
Part of systemic disease
Collagen disease
Wegener's granulomatosis
Allergic vasculitis
Temporal arteritis (see Chapter 13)

FIG. 14.2 ORBITAL INFLAMMATION
(SEE CHAPTERS 3 AND 4)

Acute
Nonsuppurative
Suppurative
Purulent infection
Phycomycosis (mucormycosis)
Chronic
Nongranulomatous
Granulomatous

FIG. 14.5 OCULAR MUSCLE INVOLVEMENT IN SYSTEMIC DISEASES

Graves' disease
Myasthenia gravis
Myotonia dystrophica
Collagen diseases
Sarcoidosis
Trichinosis
Primary amyloidosis

FIG. 14.6 GRAVES' DISEASE

Mild
Onset early in adult life
Affects predominantly women
Bilateral (may initially be unilateral)
Ocular proptosis nil to mild to moderate (lid retraction often simulates exophthalmos)
Prognosis for vision good

Severe
Onset in middle age (average: 50 years)
Affects both sexes equally (except postthyroidectomy, when men predominate 4:1)
Bilateral (may initially be unilateral)
Severe proptosis
Poor visual prognosis
The patient may be hypothyroid, hyperthyroid, or euthyroid

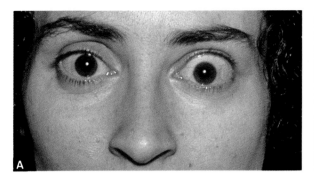

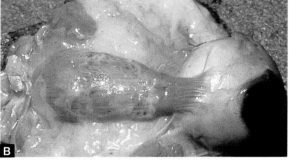

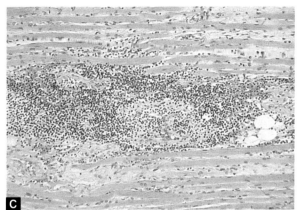

Fig. 14.7 Graves' Disease. A Most of the time, the exophthalmos in Graves' disease is more apparent than real, because of the extreme lid retraction that may occur. This patient, for instance, had minimal proptosis of the left eye but marked lid retraction. **B** The orbital contents obtained postmortem from a patient with Graves' disease. Note the enormously thickened extraocular muscle. **C** A histologic section shows both fluid and inflammatory cells separating the muscle bundles. The inflammatory cells are predominantly lymphocytes plus plasma cells. (**A** courtesy of Dr. HG Scheie; **B**, **C**, courtesy of Dr. RC Eagle, Jr and reported by Hufnagel TJ, et al: Ophthalmology 91:1411, 1984.)

FIG. 14.8 CLASSIFICATION OF ORBITAL TUMORS

Primary in orbit   **Direct extension**
Choristomas   **Metastatic from distant sites**
Hamartomas
Mesenchymal
Neural
Lymphoid and inflammatory
Epithelial (lacrimal gland)

FIG. 14.9 CHORISTOMAS

Dermoid   Teratoma
Epidermoid   Ectopic lacrimal gland

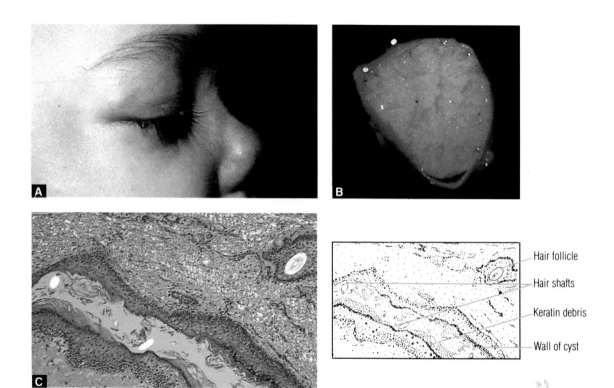

Fig. 14.10 **Dermoid. A** A dermoid tumor is present in its most common location, i.e., the superior temporal portion of the orbit. **B** Gross examination of the cut surface of the tumor shows a cyst filled with "cheesy" material. **C** A histologic section, viewed using polarized light, shows a cyst lined by stratified squamous epithelium. Hair follicles (which contain birefringent hair shafts) and other epidermal appendages are contained in the wall of the cyst. The cyst itself contains keratin debris and hair shafts which are birefringent in the polarized light. (**A**, courtesy of Dr. JA Katowitz; **B**, from *Ocular Pathology*, 2nd edn, by M Yanoff and BS Fine.)

FIG. 14.11 HAMARTOMAS

Lymphangioma

Hemangioma

Hemangiosarcoma

Hemangiopericytoma

Kaposi's sarcoma [especially associated with acquired immune deficiency syndrome (AIDS)]

Phacomatoses (see Chapter 2)

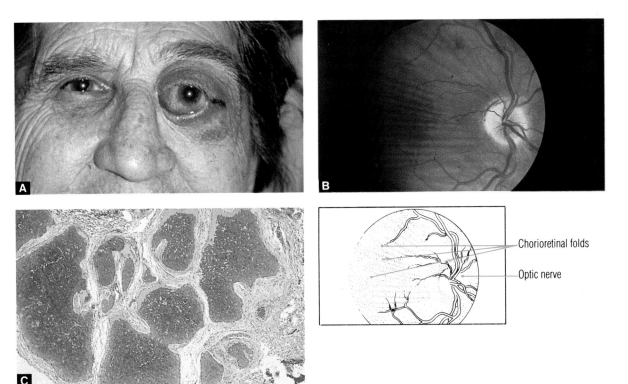

Fig. 14.12 Hemangioma. A The patient had increasing proptosis of the left eye. Even though a hemangioma is a congenital tumor, the increase in size often does not occur until adult life because of hemorrhage into the tumor or inflammatory changes.

B Another case shows that the orbital hemangioma has caused chorioretinal folds. **C** A histologic section shows large, blood-filled spaces, lined by endothelium. The septa between the blood channels are of differing thicknesses. (**A**, **B**, courtesy of Dr. HG Scheie.)

FIG. 14.13 MESENCHYMAL TUMORS

Lipoma*, liposarcoma*

Fibroma*, fibrosarcoma*

Fibrous histiocytoma

Chondroma*, chondrosarcoma*

Osteoma*, osteosarcoma*

Leiomyoma*, leiomyosarcoma*

Rhabdomyoma*, rhabdomyosarcoma

*Rare except following radiation therapy

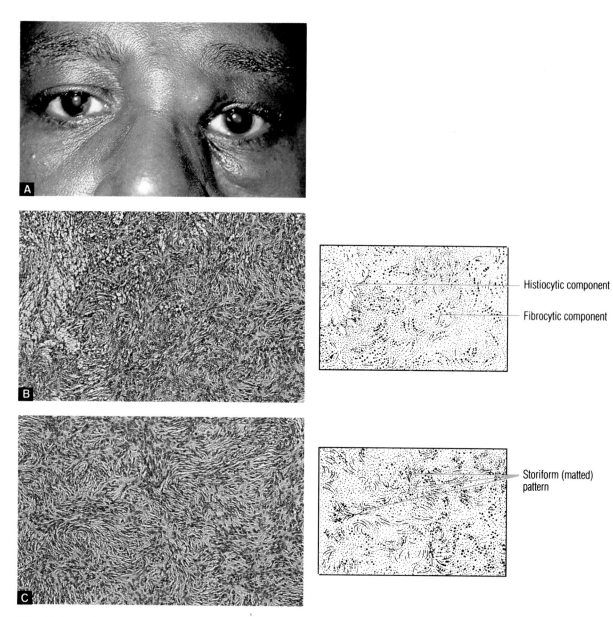

Histiocytic component

Fibrocytic component

Storiform (matted) pattern

Fig. 14.14 Fibrous Histiocytoma. A This is the fourth recurrence of an orbital tumor that first had been excised 10 years previously. The histology of the primary lesion and of the four recurrences all appear identical. **B** A histologic section shows the diphasic pattern consisting of an histiocytic component and a fibrous component. **C** Increased magnification shows that the fibrous component forms a storiform or matted pattern. Controversy exists as to whether the tumor arises from histiocytes or fibroblasts (most of the evidence points towards a fibroblastic origin). (Case reported by Jones WD, et al: Br J Plast Surg 32:46, 1979.)

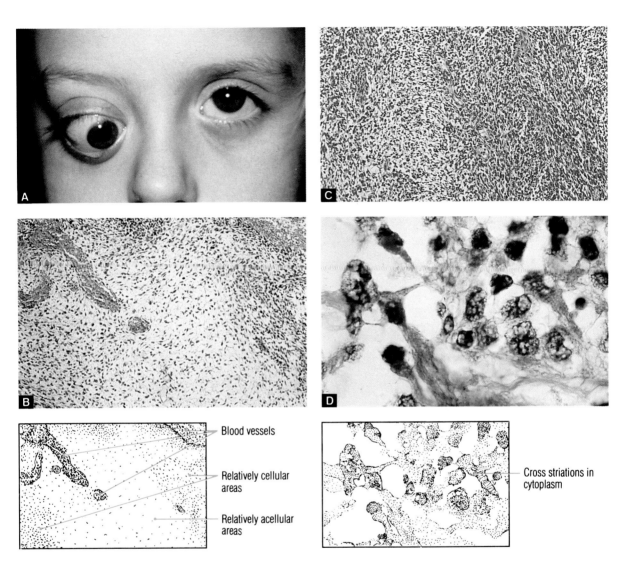

Fig. 14.15 Rhabdomyosarcoma. A The patient has a unilateral proptosis of very recent onset. Often, rhabdomyosarcoma presents rapidly, causes lid redness, and is mistaken for orbital inflammation. **B** A histologic section shows a marked embryonic cellular pattern, hence the term embryonal rhabdomyosarcoma. **C** Increased magnification shows the primitive nature of the rhabdomyoblasts; these tend to cluster in groups, separated by relatively acellular areas. **D** A trichrome stain shows characteristic cross striations in the cytoplasm of some of the rhabdomyoblasts. Cross striations, although not abundant in embryonal rhabdomyosarcoma, can be seen in sections stained with hematoxylin and eosin, but they are easier to see with special stains.

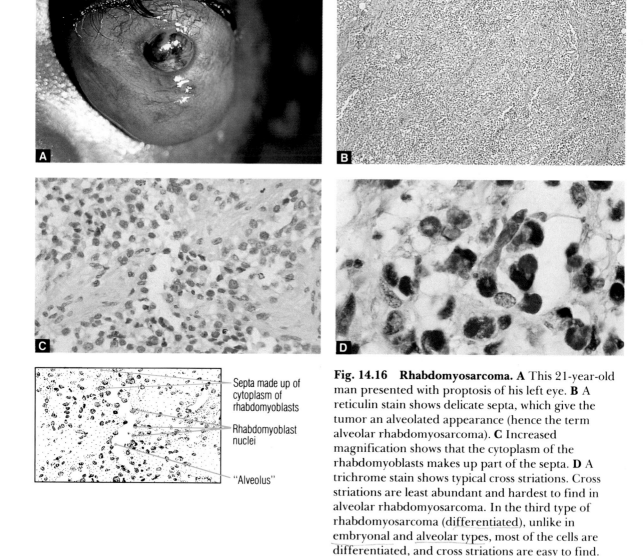

Septa made up of
cytoplasm of
rhabdomyoblasts

Rhabdomyoblast
nuclei

"Alveolus"

Fig. 14.16   Rhabdomyosarcoma. A This 21-year-old
man presented with proptosis of his left eye. **B** A
reticulin stain shows delicate septa, which give the
tumor an alveolated appearance (hence the term
alveolar rhabdomyosarcoma). **C** Increased
magnification shows that the cytoplasm of the
rhabdomyoblasts makes up part of the septa. **D** A
trichrome stain shows typical cross striations. Cross
striations are least abundant and hardest to find in
alveolar rhabdomyosarcoma. In the third type of
rhabdomyosarcoma (differentiated), unlike in
embryonal and alveolar types, most of the cells are
differentiated, and cross striations are easy to find.

FIG. 14.17 NEURAL TUMORS	
Amputation neuroma	Meningioma (see Chapter 13)
Neurofibroma (see Chapter 2)	Nonchromaffin paraganglioma (cartoid body
Neurilemmoma (schwannoma)	tumor)
Juvenile pilocytic astrocytoma (glioma) of optic	Granular cell tumor
nerve (see Chapter 13)	Alveolar soft part sarcoma

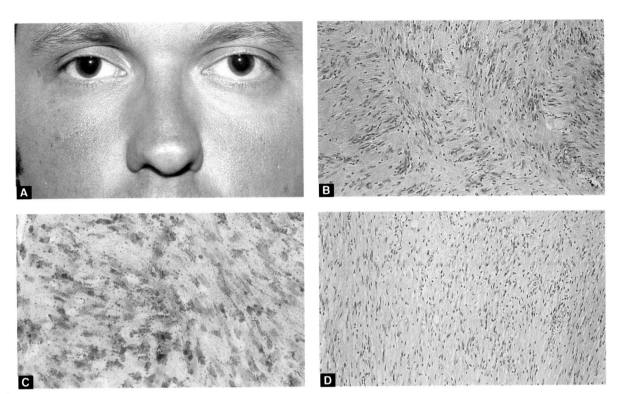

Fig. 14.18 Neurilemmoma. A Proptosis of the patient's left eye had been present for many months and was increasing in size. An orbital tumor was removed. **B** A histologic section shows ribbons of spindle Schwann cell nuclei, which show a tendency toward palisading. Areas of relative acellularity, mimicking tactile corpuscles, are called Verocay bodies. This pattern is called the Antoni type A pattern. **C** Oil red-O stain shows the cytoplasm of the tumor cells is quite lipid positive. **D** In this area of necrosis, inflammatory cells and microcystoid degeneration are present. This degenerative pattern is called the Antoni type B pattern.

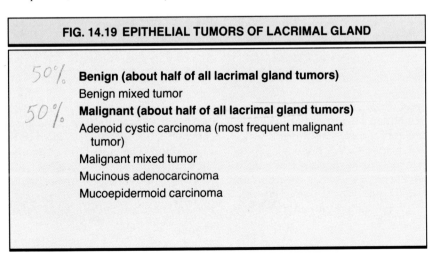

FIG. 14.19 EPITHELIAL TUMORS OF LACRIMAL GLAND

50%
Benign (about half of all lacrimal gland tumors)
Benign mixed tumor

50%
Malignant (about half of all lacrimal gland tumors)
Adenoid cystic carcinoma (most frequent malignant tumor)
Malignant mixed tumor
Mucinous adenocarcinoma
Mucoepidermoid carcinoma

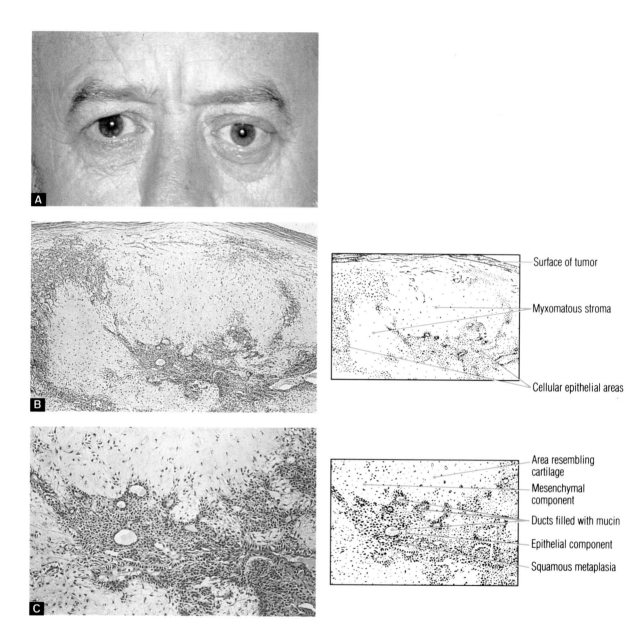

Surface of tumor

Myxomatous stroma

Cellular epithelial areas

Area resembling cartilage

Mesenchymal component

Ducts filled with mucin

Epithelial component

Squamous metaplasia

Fig. 14.20   Benign Mixed Tumor. A The patient had proptosis of the left eye for quite some time. It had gradually increased in severity. **B** A histologic section shows the characteristic diphasic pattern consisting of a pale background that has a myxomatous stroma and a relatively amorphous appearance, contiguous with quite cellular areas that contain mainly epithelial cells.

C Increased magnification shows the characteristic, epithelial, ductal structures lined by two layers of epithelium. The outer layer often undergoes myxoid and even cartilaginous metaplasia, whereas the inner layer may secrete mucus or may undergo squamous metaplasia, both of which are present here. (**A,** from *Ocular Pathology,* 2nd edn, by M Yanoff and BS Fine.)

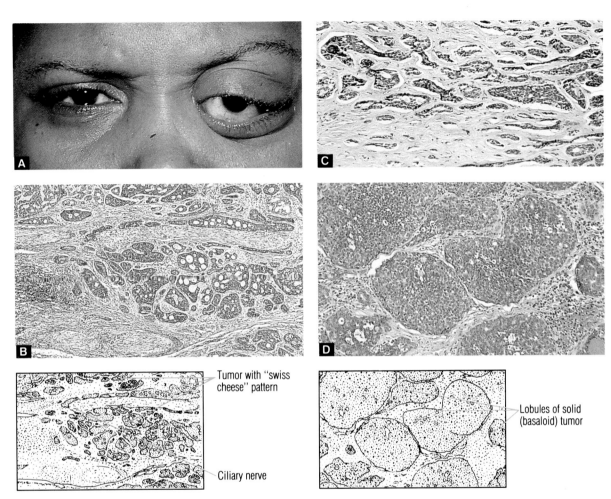

Fig. 14.21   Adenoid Cystic Carcinoma. A The patient had a rapidly progressing proptosis of the left eye. **B** A histologic section shows the characteristic, swiss cheese pattern of adenoid cystic carcinoma. The tumor is present in the perineural sheath around a ciliary nerve. Adenoid cystic carcinoma is noted for its rapid invasion of ciliary nerves. **C** The tumor may superficially resemble a basal cell carcinoma, but it tends to have a relatively acellular, hyalin-like stroma between the islands of poorly differentiated, tightly packed, small, dark epithelial cells. A basal cell carcinoma tends to have a very cellular, desmoplastic stroma between the nests of malignant basal cells. **D** In this area, a more solid pattern (basaloid pattern) is seen. This type of pattern is present in about 50% of tumors. If no basaloid pattern is seen, the 5-year survival rate is 70%; when a basaloid pattern is noted, the 5-year survival rate is 20%. (**A, B**, from *Ocular Pathology*, 2nd edn, by M Yanoff and BS Fine.)

FIG. 14.22   LESIONS OF THE IMMUNE SYSTEM

Inflammatory pseudotumor	Malignant lymphoma and leukemia
Benign lymphoid hyperplasia	Sinus histiocytosis

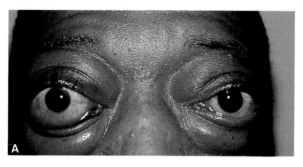

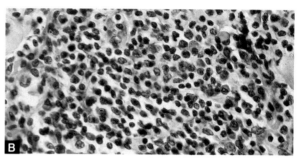

Fig. 14.23 Inflammatory Pseudotumor. A A 45-year-old man has bilateral exophthalmos, which is much worse in the right eye. **B** A biopsy of the right orbital tumor shows a mixed inflammatory infiltrate of lymphocytes, plasma cells, and histiocytes. Other sections showed lymphoid follicles which contained germinal centers, and young budding capillaries. This pattern is characteristic of an inflammatory pseudotumor. Histologically, cases like this are easy to diagnose as inflammatory. (**A,** from *Ocular Pathology,* 2nd edn, by M Yanoff and BS Fine.)

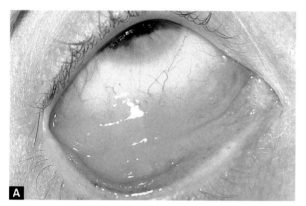

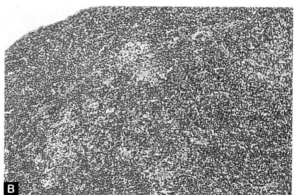

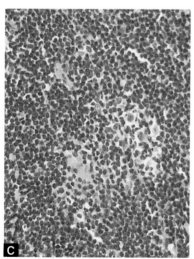

Fig. 14.24 Benign Lymphoid Hyperplasia. A The patient noted a fullness of the lower right lid. Large, thickened, redundant folds of conjunctiva in the inferior cul de sac are seen. The conjunctival lesion has a characteristic fish-flesh appearance and contains few blood vessels. The clinical differential diagnosis here is between a lymphoid lesion and amyloidosis. **B** A histologic section shows a lymphoid infiltrate. **C** Increased magnification shows that the lymphocytes are mature, quite small, and uniform; occasional plasma cells and large histiocytes are seen. The monotonous appearance of lymphocytes makes it difficult to differentiate this benign lesion from a well differentiated lymphosarcoma. The very mature appearance of the cells and the absence of atypical cells, along with the presence of plasma cells, helps to make the diagnosis of a benign lesion. In such cases, testing using monoclonal antibodies may be quite helpful. If the population is a mixed population of B and T cells, the chances are that the tumor is benign. If it is predominantly of one cell type or the other, it is probably malignant. (**A,** from *Ocular Pathology,* 2nd edn, by M Yanoff and BS Fine.)

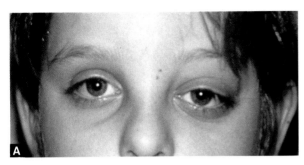

Fig. 14.25 Leukemia. A A 9-year-old boy presented with a drooping left upper lid and proptosis of the left eye. A painless left orbital mass was found. The work-up, including a complete blood count, showed normal results. He had no other signs or symptoms. An orbital biopsy was performed. **B** A histologic section shows a diffuse cellular infiltrate of primitive granulocytic leukemic cells. **C** Because of the findings in the orbital biopsy, a bone marrow aspirate was obtained. The smear shows blast cells. In most malignant lymphomas and leukemias, the atypical cell types make the diagnosis of malignancy relatively easy. (**A** from *Ocular Pathology*, 2nd edn, by M Yanoff and BS Fine.)

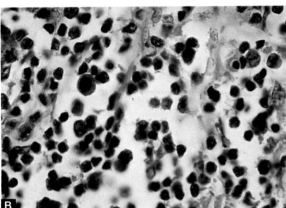

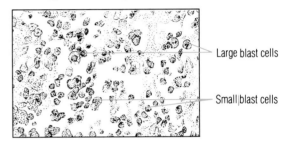

Large blast cells

Small blast cells

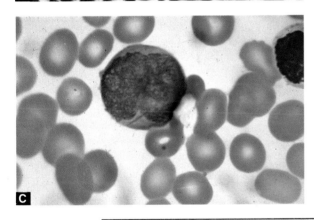

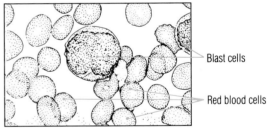

Blast cells

Red blood cells

FIG. 14.26   ORBITAL TUMORS RELATED TO SYSTEMIC DISEASE

Langerhans' cell granulomatosis (histiocytosis X)

Fibrous dysplasia

Juvenile fibromatosis

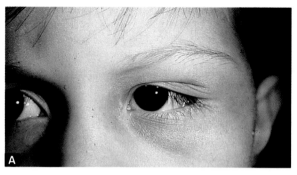

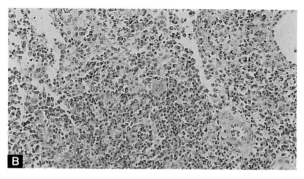

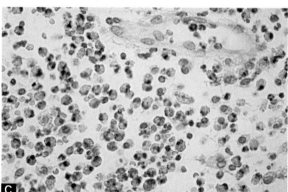

Fig. 14.27 **Eosinophilic Granuloma. A** This 4-year-old boy presented clinically with a rapid onset of erythema and swelling over the lateral edge of his orbit. Osteomyelitis or rhabdomyosarcoma were diagnosed. A biopsy was performed. **B** A histologic section shows numerous large, abnormal, histiocytes and many eosinophils. **C** Increased magnification shows the abnormal histiocytes, which contain pale cytoplasm and large, vesicular nuclei along with many eosinophils. Eosinophilic granuloma is classified within the group of Langerhans' cell granulomatosis (histiocytosis X). (**A** from *Ocular Pathology*, 2nd edn, by M Yanoff and BS Fine.)

FIG. 14.28   SECONDARY ORBITAL TUMORS

Direct extension
Malignant melanoma of uvea, conjunctiva, or lid
Retinoblastoma
Squamous cell carcinoma of conjunctiva
Basal cell carcinoma of lid
Sebaceous gland carcinoma of lid
Tumors of the upper respiratory tract
Tumors of the nasolacrimal apparatus
Meningioma

Metastatic from distant sites
Breast
Lung
Adrenal (neuroblastoma)
Pancreas
Others

Bibliography

Ellis JH, et al: Lymphoid tumors of the ocular adnexa. Clinical correlation with the working formulation classification and immunoperoxidase staining of paraffin sections. Ophthalmology 92:1311, 1985.

Feldman RB, et al: Solitary eosinophilic granuloma of the lateral orbital wall. Am J Ophthalmol 100:318, 1985.

Feldon SE, Muramatsu S, Weiner JM: Clinical classification of Graves' ophthalmopathy. Identification of risk factors for optic neuropathy. Arch Ophthalmol 102:1469, 1984.

Font RL, Hidayat AA: Fibrous histiocytoma of the orbit. A clinicopathologic study of 150 cases. Hum Pathol 13:199, 1982.

Hufnagel TJ, et al: Immunohistochemical and ultrastructural studies on the exenterated orbital tissues of a patient with Graves' disease. Ophthalmology 91:1411, 1984.

Iwamoto T, Jakobiec FA: A comparative ultrastructural study of the normal lacrimal gland and its epithelial tumors. Hum Pathol 13:236, 1982.

Johnson LN, et al: Sinus tumors invading the orbit. Ophthalmology 91:209, 1984.

Jones WD III, Yanoff M, Katowitz JA: Recurrent facial fibrous histiocytoma. Br J Plast Surg 32:46, 1975.

Knowles DM II, Jakobiec FA: Ocular adnexal lymphoid neoplasms: clinical, histopathologic, electron microsopic, and immunologic characteristics. Hum Pathol 13:148, 1982.

Lazzarino M, et al: Clinicopathologic and immunologic characteristics of non-Hodgkin's lymphomas presenting in the orbit. Cancer 55:1907, 1985.

Lee DA, et al: A clinicopathologic study of primary adenoid cystic carcinoma of the lacrimal gland. Ophthalmology 92:128, 1985.

Ruchman MC, Flanagan J: Cavernous hemangioma of the orbit. Ophthalmology 90:1328, 1983.

Sergott RC, Glaser JS: Graves' ophthalmopathy. A clinical and immunologic review. (Review). Surv Ophthalmol 26:1, 1981.

Shields JA, et al: Classification and incidence of space occupying lesions of the orbit. A survey of 645 biopsies. Arch Ophthalmol 102:1606, 1984.

Zimmerman RA, et al: Orbital magnetic resonance imaging. Am J Ophthalmol 100:312, 1985.

DIABETES MELLITUS 15

Diabetic retinopathy currently is the leading cause of blindness in adults under the age of 65. In addition, diabetic retinopathy is the second leading cause of new blindness each year. Approximately 70% of those who have had diabetes mellitus for more than 10 years will develop retinopathy. In fewer than 10% of these cases, however, will the retinopathy progress to blindness.

Diabetes affects many ocular structures. Major effects may be seen clinically and histologically, in the retina as diabetic retinopathy, and in the iris as neovascularization of the stroma and vacuolization of the pigment epithelium. Other significant changes may be seen histologically in the ciliary body (thickened basement membrane) and in the choroid (diabetic choroidopathy). It is unclear whether or not diabetics show an earlier or an increased incidence of cataract development. The optic nerve may be involved in neovascularization or in ischemic (nonarteritic) optic neuropathy.

FIG. 15.1 BACKGROUND DIABETIC RETINOPATHY
—A CONSTELLATION OF FINDINGS

Microaneurysms	Exudates
Edema	Hemorrhages

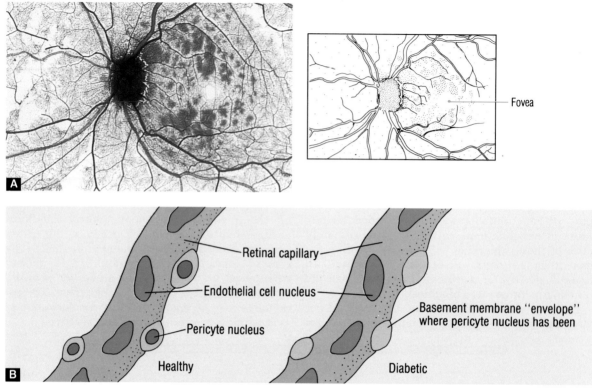

Fovea

Retinal capillary

Endothelial cell nucleus

Basement membrane "envelope" where pericyte nucleus has been

Pericyte nucleus

Healthy

Diabetic

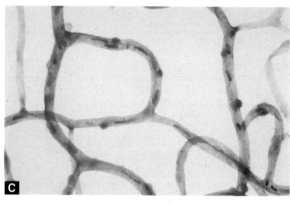

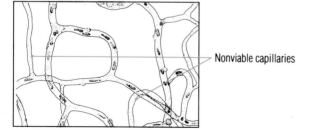

Nonviable capillaries

Fig. 15.2   Retinal Vasculature (Normal and Diabetic). A The trypsin-digest preparation of the retina, stained with PAS and hematoxylin, shows the optic nerve and the major retinal blood vessels. The capillary-free zone of the fovea is seen clearly. **B** In a retinal capillary of a normal eye the ratio of pericyte nuclei to endothelial cell nuclei is 1:1. In a diabetic, the ratio is decreased because of a drop-out of pericyte nuclei. The normal endothelial cell cytoplasm, covered externally by a basement membrane, makes up the wall of the retinal capillary. The normal pericyte nucleus sits as a button on the surface of the capillary and sends cytoplasmic processes, in a discontinuous fashion, around the capillary. The normal pericyte is completely surrounded by basement membrane (basement membrane envelope). **C** In capillaries of diabetic patients, the basement membrane envelopes no longer contain pericyte nuclei and are themselves thickened by PAS-positive material. The endothelial cells, although somewhat pyknotic, remain in relatively normal numbers.

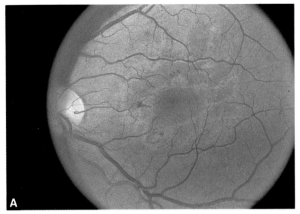

Fig. 15.3   Retinal Capillary Microaneurysm.
A Background diabetic retinopathy consists of retinal capillary microaneurysms (RCMs), hemorrhages, edema, and exudates. In this fundus photograph a RCM and a tiny hemorrhage are seen. **B** Trypsin digest shows that a RCM consists of a proliferation of endothelial cells. **C** A histologic section shows a large, blood filled space, lined by endothelium. The caliber is about that of a venule. Venules, however, do not occur in this location (in the inner nuclear layer), but are found mainly in the nerve fiber layer. By a process of elimination, therefore, we know that we are looking at a cross section of a RCM. (**A**, **C**, from *Ocular Pathology*, 2nd edn, by M Yanoff and BS Fine.)

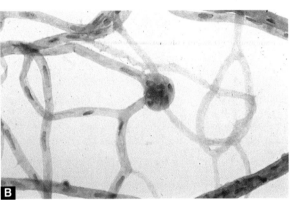

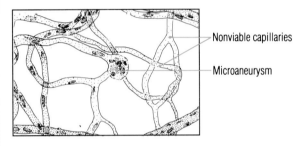

Nonviable capillaries

Microaneurysm

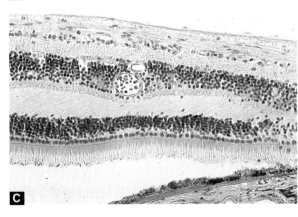

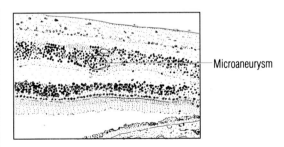

Microaneurysm

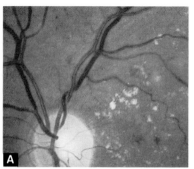

Fig. 15.4 Exudates. A Scattered, hard, waxy exudates are seen. **B** A histologic section of another case shows a collection of eosinophilic material in the outer plexiform layer, the characteristic location of diabetic exudates. The nuclei within the fluid represent histiocytes. **C** A thin section of a plastic-embedded retina shows collections of fluid within the outer plexiform layer. In some areas, the exudate is occupied completely by histiocytes. **D** Oil red-O shows that the material within the exudates stains positive (red) (**A, B**, from *Ocular Pathology*, 2nd edn, by M Yanoff and BS Fine.)

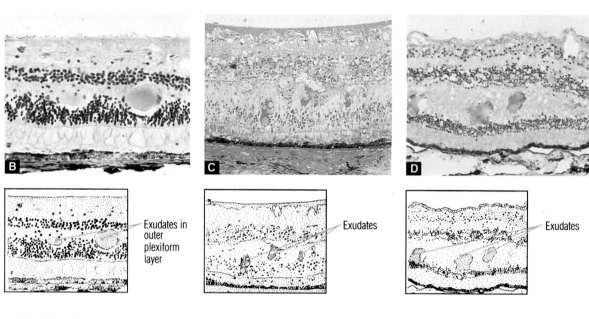

Exudates in outer plexiform layer

Exudates

Exudates

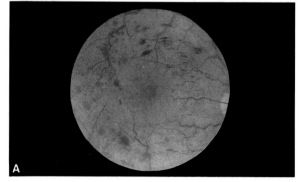

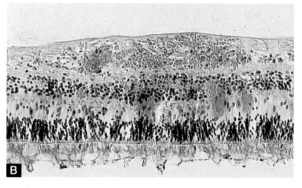

Fig. 15.5 Hemorrhagic Retinopathy. A Dot, blot, flame-shaped, and globular hemorrhages are present within the retina. **B** Flame-shaped or splinter hemorrhages consist of small collections of blood in the nerve fiber layer. Dot and blot hemorrhages are caused by small hemorrhagic collections in the inner nuclear and outer plexiform layers. (**A**, from *Ocular Pathology*, 2nd edn, by M Yanoff and BS Fine.)

FIG. 15.6 PREPROLIFERATIVE RETINOPATHY—A CONSTELLATION OF FINDINGS

Cotton wool spots	Intraretinal microvascular abnormalities (IRMA)
Venous beading	Increasing retinal hemorrhages

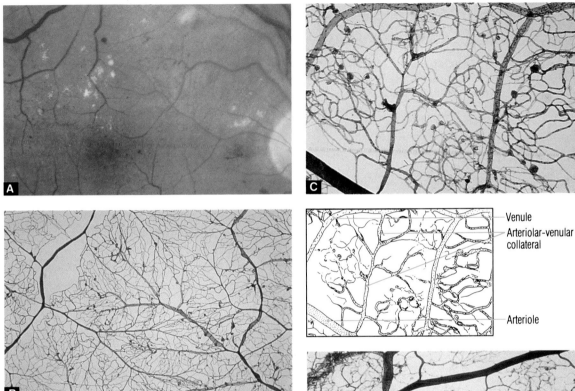

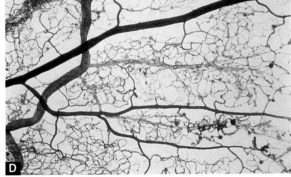

Venule
Arteriolar-venular collateral

Arteriole

Fig. 15.7   Preproliferative Retinopathy. A A cotton wool spot of recent onset is present just inferior to the superior arcade. **B** Trypsin-digest preparation shows sausage-shaped dilated venules. **C** An arteriolar–venular collateral vessel is present. **D** Intraretinal microvascular abnormalities (IRMA) are present in the form of dilated capillaries, capillary buds and loops, and areas of capillary closure.

FIG. 15.8 PROLIFERATIVE RETINOPATHY

Pure neovascularization	Fibrovascular membranes	Retinal detachment

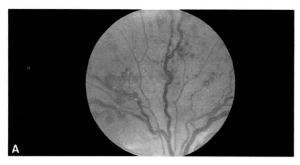

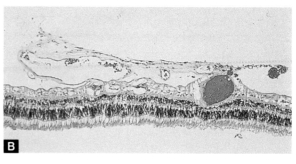

Fig. 15.9 Neovascularization. A The superior venule is dilated and beaded. Neovascular tufts are arising from venules. **B** A histologic section of another case shows new blood vessels arising from a retinal venule, perforating the internal limiting membrane, and spreading out on the internal surface of the retina, between the internal limiting membrane and the vitreous body. In this location, the new, abnormal, fragile blood vessels may be subject to trauma (e.g., vitreous detachment) and result in a subvitreal hemorrhage between the retinal internal limiting membrane and the posterior hyaloid of the separated vitreous body. (**A**, from *Ocular Pathology*, 2nd edn, by M Yanoff and BS Fine.)

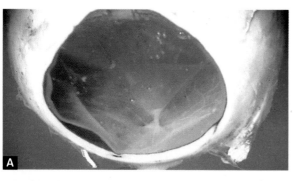

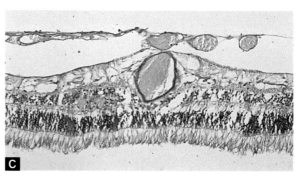

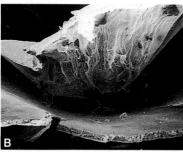

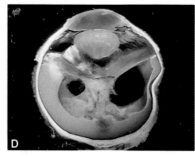

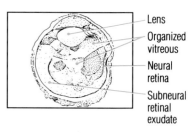

Fig. 15.10 Neovascularization. A A tuft of neovascularization arising from the optic nerve head is attached to the posterior surface of an otherwise detached vitreous body. **B** Scanning electron microscopy shows blood vessels arising from the internal surface of the retina and attaching to the posterior surface of the partially detached vitreous. **C** A PAS-stained, histologic section shows blood vessels originating from a retinal venule and attaching to the posterior surface of the vitreous. **D** The gross specimen shows the end stage of diabetic retinopathy. Extensive neovascularization of the retina and the detached vitreous have resulted in a traction retinal detachment. The subretinal space is filled with a gelatinous material. (**B**, courtesy of Dr. RC Eagle Jr.; **D**, from *Ocular Pathology*, 2nd edn, by M Yanoff and BS Fine.)

FIG. 15.11 DIABETIC CHANGES IN IRIS, CHOROID, AND CILIARY BODY

Diabetic iridopathy
Neovascularization
Lacy vacuolization

Diabetic choroidopathy
Occlusion of the choriocapillaris
Thickening (hyperproduction)
    of vascular basement membranes
Arteriolarsclerosis

Diabetic changes in the ciliary body
Diffuse thickening of outer
    basement membrane

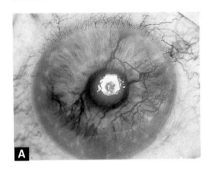

Fig. 15.12 Iris neovascularization. A The patient shows neovascularization of the iris. Clinically, the reddish appearance of the iris, caused by the abnormal anterior surface blood vessels, is called rubeosis iridis. **B** A histologic section of another case shows a peripheral anterior synechia and a thick mantle of tissue anterior to the pigmented anterior border layer of the iris. The tissue is fibrovascular tissue. Contraction of the tissue has caused an eversion of the iris pigment epithelium and sphincter muscle. This eversion is called ectropion uveae. Tissue anterior to the normally avascular anterior border layer of the iris usually signifies neovascularization (as in this case), inflammation, or neoplasm. **C** In another case, a histologic section shows that the neovascularization has caused adherence between the peripheral iris and the cornea, called peripheral anterior synechia.

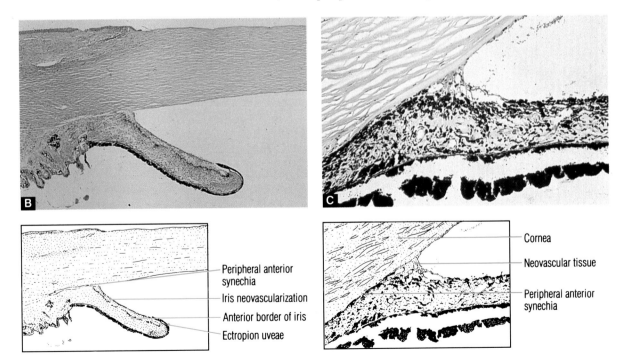

Peripheral anterior synechia
Iris neovascularization
Anterior border of iris
Ectropion uveae

Cornea
Neovascular tissue
Peripheral anterior synechia

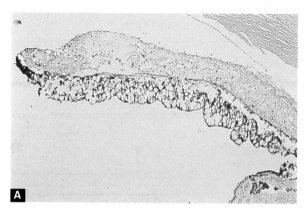

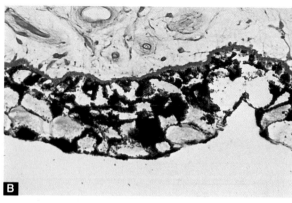

Fig. 15.13 Lacy Vacuolation of Iris Pigment Epithelium. A Large vacuoles are present in both the anterior and posterior layers of the iris pigment epithelium. The vacuoles appear empty in sections stained with hematoxylin and eosin. **B** PAS stain shows that the vacuoles contain a PAS-positive material. Pretreatment of the sections with diastase eliminates the PAS reaction, signifying that the vacuolar material is glycogen.

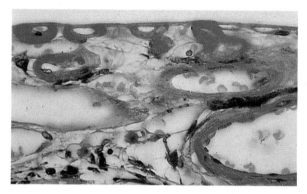

Fig. 15.14 Choroidopathy. A histologic section of the foveomacular region shows diffuse thickening of choroidal vessels by periodic acid-Schiff (PAS) positive material. The choriocapillaris is prominently involved and partially occluded. The retinal pigment epithelium is absent. (Modified from Hidayat AA, Fine BS: Ophthalmology 92:512, 1985.)

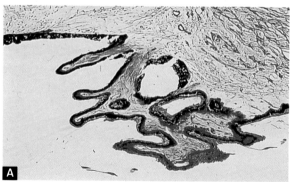

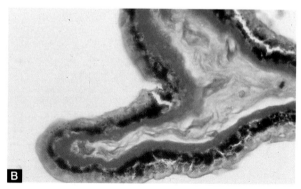

Fig. 15.15 Ciliary Body. A PAS stain shows a diffuse thickening of the basement membrane of the pigmented ciliary epithelium in the pars plicata only. **B** Increased magnification shows the thickened basement membrane. Thickening of the basement membrane of the pigmented ciliary epithelium of the pars plicata is quite characteristic of diabetes mellitus.

Bibliography

Buzney SM, et al: Retinal vascular endothelial cells and pericytes. Differential growth characteristics in vitro. Invest Ophthalmol Vis Sci 24: 470, 1983.

Frank RN: On the pathogenesis of diabetic retinopathy. Ophthalmology 91:626, 1984.

Hidayat AA, Fine BS: Diabetic choroidopathy—light and electron microscopic observations of seven cases. Ophthalmology 92:512, 1985.

Klein R, Klein BEK, Moss SE: Visual impairment in diabetes. Ophthalmology 91:1, 1984.

Miller H, et al: Diabetic neovascularization: permeability and ultrastructure. Invest Ophthalmol Vis Sci 25: 1338, 1984.

Muraoka K, Shimizu K: Intraretinal neovascularization in diabetic retinopathy. Ophthalmology 91:1440, 1984.

Niki T, Muraoka K, Shimizu K: Distribution of capillary nonperfusion in early-stage diabetic retinopathy. Ophthalmology 91:1431, 1984.

Yanoff M: Ocular pathology of diabetes mellitus. Am J Ophthalmol 67:21, 1969.

Yanoff M, Fine BS, Berkow JW: Diabetic lacy vacuolation of iris pigment epithelium. Am J Ophthalmol 69:201, 1970.

GLAUCOMA 16

Glaucoma is the leading cause of blindness among the 500,000 people legally classified as blind in the United States. Glaucoma affects:

- 0.5–1% of the population;
- 2% of people age 35 years or older;
- 3% of people age 65 years or older;
- 14% (1:7) of blind people.

Glaucoma is characterized by an intraocular pressure sufficiently elevated to produce ocular tissue damage that may be either transient or permanent. The condition is not a single disease entity; it may be primary or it may develop secondary to a variety of ocular and systemic diseases. Therefore, glaucoma is a syndrome, not an intraocular pressure reading.

A patient presenting with increased intraocular pressure without detectable ocular tissue damage or visual functional impairment may be said to have ocular hypertension or be glaucoma-suspect. Ocular hypertension may lead to ocular tissue damage, and hence to glaucoma, at an incidence of about 1% per year.

Glaucoma may be divided into two different types. One is extremely rare and is characterized by a normal outflow with hypersecretion of aqueous. The other is the common type with impaired outflow, which can be subdivided as follows:

- congenital glaucoma;
- primary open- and closed-angle glaucomas;
- secondary open- and closed-angle glaucomas.

Primary open-angle glaucoma accounts for about two-thirds of all glaucomas seen in whites, and has a prevalence between 0.5 and 1% of the population. In blacks it occurs at a rate of approximately 1.5% of the population. Primary closed-angle glaucoma occurs in less than 0.5% of the population. This type of glaucoma is much more common in whites than in blacks. However, a high percentage of blacks have the chronic, not the acute, type of closed-angle glaucoma.

FIG. 16.1 CLINICAL FEATURES OF CONGENITAL GLAUCOMA

Affects 1:5000–1:10,000 live births

Autosomal recessive

60–70% are male children

64–88% are bilateral

FIG. 16.2 CONGENITAL GLAUCOMA

Age at onset	Percentage
At birth	40
Birth–6 months	34
6 months–1 year	12
1–6 years	11
Over 6 years	2
No information	1

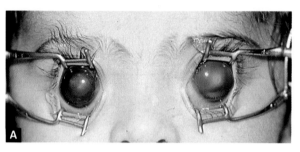

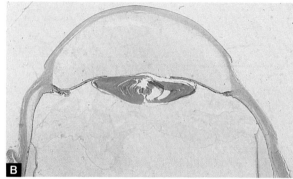

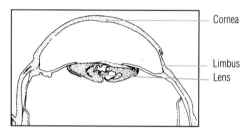

Fig. 16.4 Congenital Glaucoma. A The enlarged corneas are secondary to abnormal intraocular pressure in a patient who has congenital glaucoma, buphthalmos, and aniridia. Congenital glaucoma often presents with symptoms of tearing and photophobia. **B** In buphthalmos, enlargement of the globe is predominantly in the anterior segment and mainly in the limbal region, causing limbal ectasia. If the ectatic limbus is lined by uveal tissue in the form of iris, it is called limbal staphyloma. (**A**, courtesy of Dr. HG Scheie.)

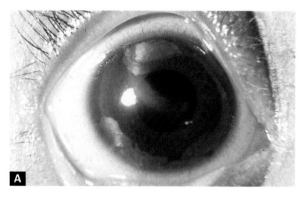

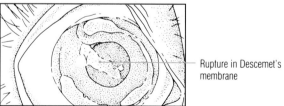

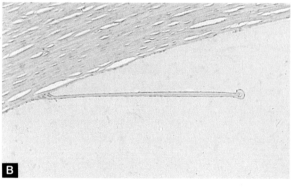

Fig. 16.5 Congenital Glaucoma. A The patient presented with congenital glaucoma and had enlarged corneas and ruptures in Descemet's membrane. **B** The ruptured ends of Descemet's membrane have sealed over. The ends, which extend into the anterior chamber, are scroll-like and covered by endothelium. (**A**, courtesy of Dr. HG Scheie.)

FIG. 16.6 CAUSES OF PRIMARY CLOSED-ANGLE GLAUCOMA

Anatomic predisposition	**Precipitating factors**
High hypermetropia	Dim light leading to middilatation
	Swelling of a cataractous lens

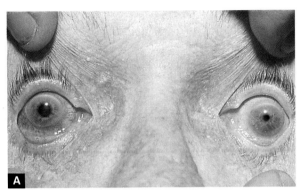

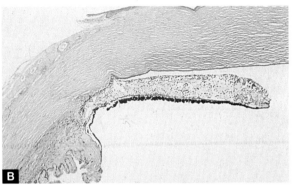

Fig. 16.7   Closed-angle Glaucoma. A The patient complained of pain, photophobia, and of seeing halos around lights. Note the semidilated pupil and the ciliary injection in the right eye. **B** The eye was removed from a patient who had closed-angle glaucoma. The anterior chamber angle is completely occluded by a peripheral anterior synechia. The iris shows segmental necrosis consisting of stromal atrophy, loss of the dilator muscle, and necrosis of the sphincter muscle. Segmental iris necrosis can be mimicked clinically by herpes zoster. (**B**, PAS.)

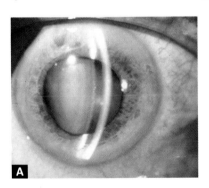

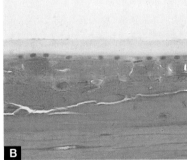

Fig. 16.8   Closed-angle Glaucoma. A Lens exhibits presence of glaukomflecken (tiny, white, anterior subcapsular lens opacities). **B** Histologic section shows small areas of epithelial necrosis in the lens, and tiny adjacent areas of subcapsular cortical degeneration. (**A**, courtesy of Dr. DM Kozart.)

FIG. 16.9 CAUSES OF PRIMARY OPEN-ANGLE GLAUCOMA

Causes and pathology unclear but seem related to acceleration of aging processes

Autosomal recessive

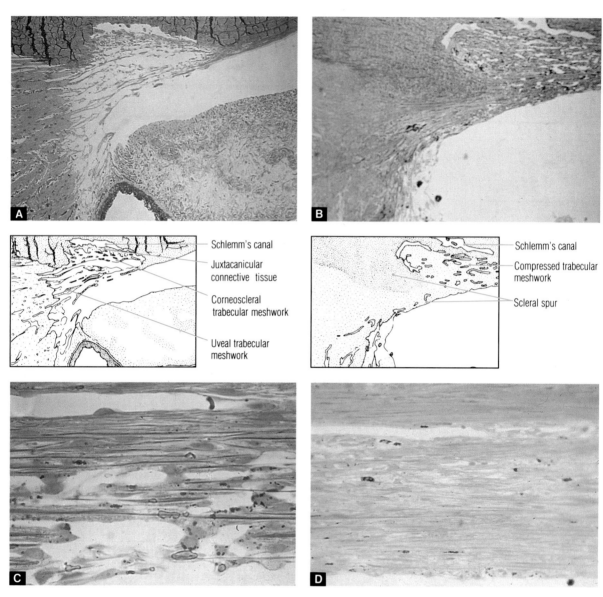

Schlemm's canal
Juxtacanicular connective tissue
Corneoscleral trabecular meshwork

Uveal trabecular meshwork

Schlemm's canal
Compressed trabecular meshwork

Scleral spur

Fig. 16.10 Open-angle Glaucoma. A The normal anterior chamber angle shows a loose arrangement of trabecular meshwork in both the corneoscleral and uveal components. The juxtacanalicular connective tissue of the trabecular meshwork is adjacent to Schlemm's canal. **B** An eye removed from a patient who had chronic open-angle glaucoma shows the results of the aging process. The normally loose tissue in the uveal trabecular meshwork and angle recess has compacted, producing a prominent scleral spur. **C** A coronal section taken through normal trabecular meshwork shows that the loose beams of the meshwork form large tubes running in an anterior–posterior direction. **D** Coronal sections through the trabecular meshwork in a patient who had chronic open-angle glaucoma show that the aging process has caused marked compaction of the beams of the trabecular meshwork, resulting in occlusion of most of the tubes, (**A, B, C,** and **D,** PD; case reported in Fine BS et al, 1981; **A,** rhesus monkey.)

FIG. 16.11 CAUSES OF SECONDARY CLOSED-ANGLE GLAUCOMA

Chronic primary closed angle	Anterior uveitis	Endo- or epithelialization
Phacomorphic lens swelling	Spherophakia	Iris neovascularization
Anterior lens dislocation	Seclusion of pupil (iris bombé)	Cysts of iris and ciliary body
Posttraumatic flat anterior chamber	Retinopathy of prematurity	Juvenile xanthogranuloma
Iridocorneal endothelial (ICE) syndrome	Persistent hyperplastic primary vitreous	Uveal melanoma

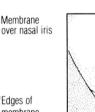
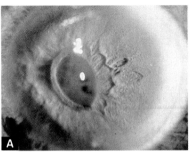
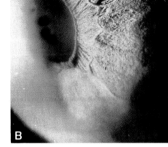
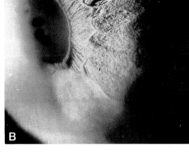
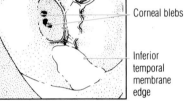

Fig. 16.12 Iridocorneal Endothelial (ICE) Syndrome (Iris Nevus Syndrome Variant). A Unilateral corneal edema and heterochromia in a patient with ICE syndrome. The temporal half of the iris is relatively normal; the nasal half shows ectropion uvea and effacement of the normal iris pattern by a membrane (probably Descemet's). **B** The inferior temporal transition zone between the normal temporal section of the iris and the membrane is seen clearly. Note corneal blebs in region of the pupil. (**A** and **B**, courtesy of Dr. DM Kozart; from *Ocular Pathology*, 2nd edn, by M Yanoff and BS Fine.)

Membrane over nasal iris

Edges of membrane

Corneal blebs

Inferior temporal membrane edge

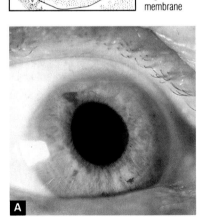

Fig. 16.13 ICE Syndrome (Iris Nevus Syndrome Variant). A Note the irregularity on the superior aspect of the pupillary margin, the dark iris nevus, and the effacement of the iris stroma superiorly. **B** An excisional biopsy of the superior iris shows deep stromal pigmentation. Bleached sections revealed that the pigmented cells are nevus cells. Traction by the nevus pulls pigment epithelium and sphincter forward, curving the iris to form an ectropion uveae. **C** At a different level, the peripheral iris has adhered to the overlying Descemet's membrane. Migration and proliferation of corneal endothelium from Descemet's membrane over the stromal bridge onto the anterior surface of the iris has occurred both centrally and peripherally, laying down a new Descemet's membrane. (**C**, PAS; case reported in Jakobiec FA et al, 1977.)

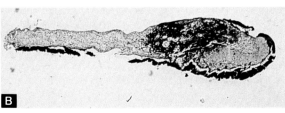
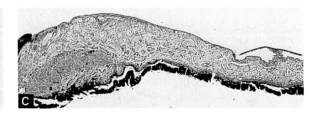

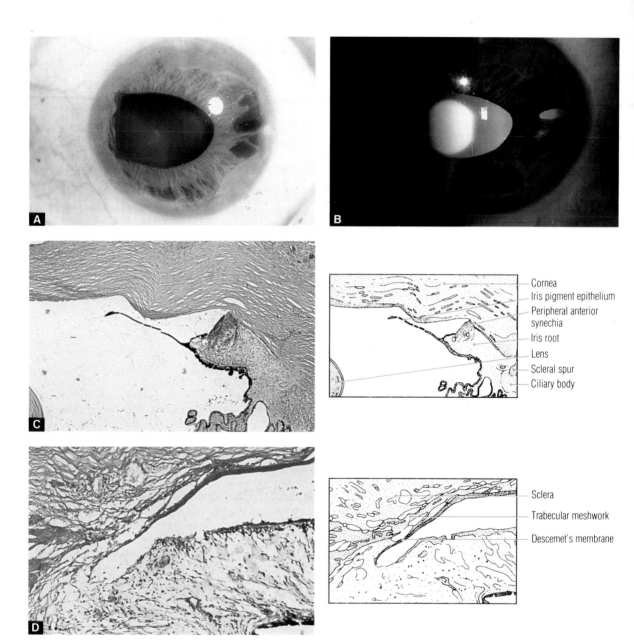

Cornea
Iris pigment epithelium
Peripheral anterior
synechia
Iris root
Lens
Scleral spur
Ciliary body

Sclera
Trabecular meshwork
Descemet's membrane

Fig. 16.14   ICE Syndrome (Essential Iris Atrophy Variant). A Slit lamp, and **B**, red reflex views of the same eye showing migration of the iris nasally toward the initial synechia, and stretching of the iris temporally, with a through-and-through iris hole. **C** Histologic section of another eye with essential iris atrophy shows a peripheral anterior synechia, marked and complete degeneration and loss of the central iris stroma, and total loss of the central iris pigment epithelium. **D** In an area away from the peripheral anterior synechia, the anterior chamber angle is open but the trabecular meshwork is covered by a proliferated corneal endothelium and Descemet's membrane. (**A** and **B**, courtesy of Dr. HG Scheie; case shown in **C** and **D** reported in Scheie HG et al, 1976.)

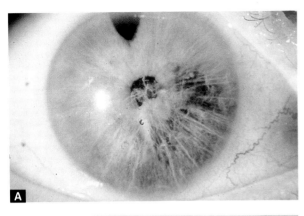

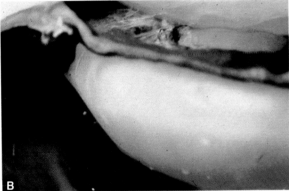

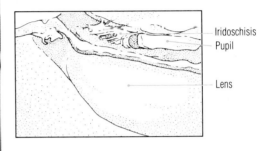

Iridoschisis
Pupil

Lens

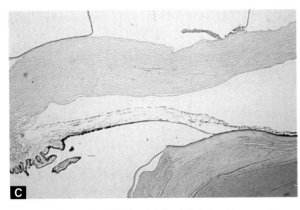

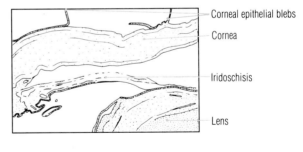

Corneal epithelial blebs

Cornea

Iridoschisis

Lens

Fig. 16.15 Iridoschisis. A The iris is in disarray in long rolled strips from the 3- to the 6-o'clock position. **B** The gross specimen from another eye shows separation and breakage of the collagenous columns of the iris stroma. **C** Histologic section of the eye shown in **B** demonstrates epithelial blebs (bullous corneal edema) and separation of the iris stroma into elongated lamellae. (**A**, courtesy of Dr. G Naumann; from *Ocular Pathology*, by M Yanoff and BS Fine.)

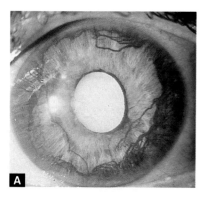

Fig. 16.16 Iris Neovascularization. A Large blood vessels growing abnormally over the anterior surface of the iris give it a reddish color, a condition called rubeosis iridis. **B** Histologic section shows vascular channels and fibrous tissue present anterior to the anterior border layer of the iris in the form of iris neovascularization. The membrane has caused a peripheral anterior synechia. Shrinkage of the membrane has produced an ectropion uveae. **C** In a scanning electron microscopic (SEM) view, the anterior chamber angle and peripheral iris are covered by a fibrovascular membrane, and the angle is closed by a peripheral anterior synechia. (**B**, PAS; **C**, SEM; **C**, courtesy of Drs. RC Eagle Jr and JW Sassani.)

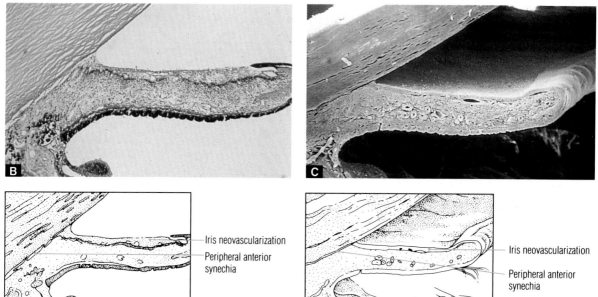

Iris neovascularization
Peripheral anterior synechia

Iris neovascularization
Peripheral anterior synechia

FIG. 16.17 CAUSES OF SECONDARY OPEN-ANGLE GLAUCOMA

Cells or debris in angle	Damaged outflow channels	Corneoscleral and extraocular conditions
Hyphema	Old uveitis	Interstitial keratitis
Uveitis	Recurrent attacks of closed-angle glaucoma	Orbital venous thrombosis
Phacolytic, hemolytic (ghost cell) and melanomalytic glaucoma	Repeated hyphema	Cavernous sinus thrombosis
Nondenatured lens material from ruptured lens	Siderosis and hemosiderosis bulbi	Carotid-cavernous fistula
Pigment dispersion syndrome	Trauma	Post retinal detachment surgery
Exfoliation syndrome	Cornea guttata	Retrobulbar mass
Uveal melanoma	Early iris neovascularization	Leukemia
Endo- or epithelialization	**Unknown mechanisms**	Mediastinal mass
	Steroids	
	α-chymotrypsin	

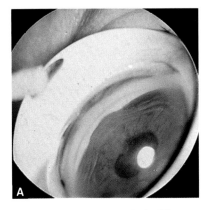

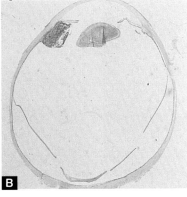

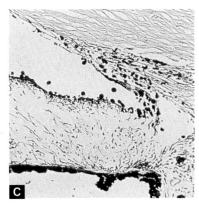

Fig. 16.18 Melanomalytic Glaucoma. A The patient presented with a markedly elevated intraocular pressure, ocular pain, and was seeing halos around lights. The angle, however, was wide open except where it was closed by a pigmented tumor, between the 8- and the 9-o'clock position. **B** The enucleated eye shows a small and completely necrotic ciliary-body melanoma. **C** Pigmented cells are seen over the anterior surface of the iris, the angle recess, and the trabecular meshwork. A bleached section of the pigmented cells showed that they are macrophages filled with pigment. The necrotic cells of the ciliary-body melanoma have lysed and liberated their melanin pigment, which has been phagocytosed by macrophages and carried by the aqueous into the anterior chamber and angle. This is analogous to what happens in phacolytic and hemolytic (ghost cell) glaucomas. (**A**, courtesy of Dr. HG Scheie; case reported in Yanoff M and Scheie HG, 1970.)

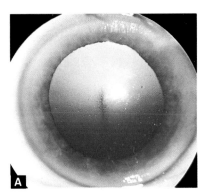

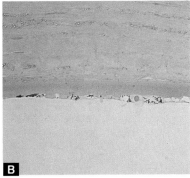

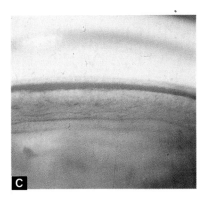

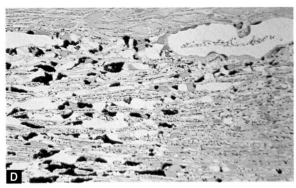

Fig. 16.19 Pigment Dispersion Syndrome. A A Krukenberg spindle is seen as a vertical linear deposition of melanin pigment in the central inferior cornea. **B** Granules of melanin pigment are present within corneal endothelial cells. **C** The anterior chamber angle is deeply pigmented. **D** Melanin pigment is present within the endothelial cells lining the beams of the trabecular meshwork.

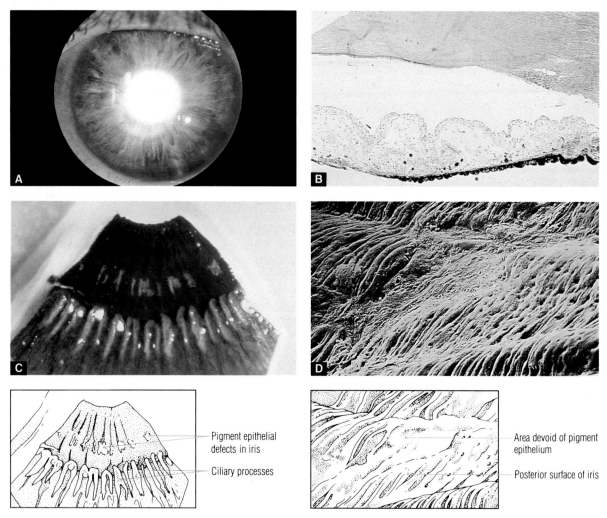

Fig. 16.20   Pigment Dispersion Syndrome.
A Extensive increased iris transillumination is present predominantly in the middle third of the iris. **B** The area of increased transillumination corresponds to the area of loss of pigment epithelium from the back of the iris. **C** The gross specimen shows loss of pigment epithelium from the back of the iris, which is seen more clearly in **D**, the SEM view of the posterior surface of the iris.

Pigment epithelial defects in iris

Ciliary processes

Area devoid of pigment epithelium

Posterior surface of iris

FIG. 16.21 MAJOR TISSUE CHANGES SECONDARY TO GLAUCOMA	
Corneal edema	Optic nerve atrophy and cupping
Degeneration of inner retinal layers	Cavernous (Schnabel's) optic atrophy

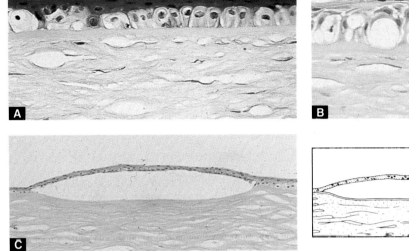

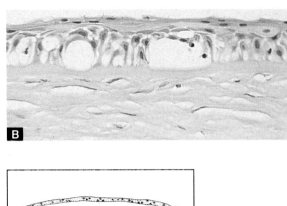

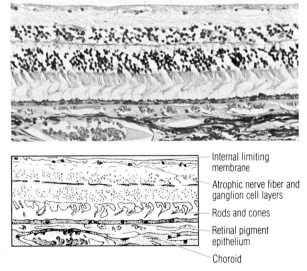

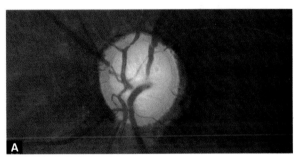

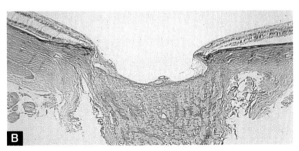

Fig. 16.22 Corneal Edema. A Fluid present in the basal layer of the corneal epithelium causes swelling of the cells. Clinically, this would appear as bedewing. **B** The edema has spread both within and between the epithelial cells. **C** Further collection of fluid has caused the entire epithelium to lift off of the Bowman's membrane, forming a large bleb. (**A**, trichrome.)

Bowman's membrane

Internal limiting membrane

Atrophic nerve fiber and ganglion cell layers

Rods and cones

Retinal pigment epithelium

Choroid

Fig. 16.23 Glaucomatous Atrophy of the Retina. As a result of glaucoma, marked atrophy of the inner layers of the retina has occurred, especially of the nerve fiber layer, which shows thinning, and of the ganglion cell layer, which shows only occasional nuclei instead of the normal continuous single layer in this nasal area.

Fig. 16.24 Optic Nerve Cupping. A Excavation of the head of the optic nerve in a patient who has chronic open-angle glaucoma. **B** The optic nerve head is deeply cupped. (**A**, courtesy of Dr. DM Kozart.)

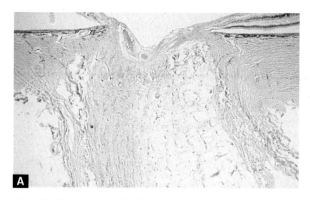

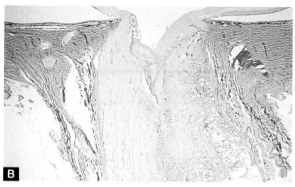

Fig. 16.25 Schnabel's Cavernous Optic Atrophy.
A The optic nerve head shows cupping of its surface and large cystic spaces in its parenchyma. **B** Special stain to test for the presence of acid mucopolysaccharides (AMP) shows that the cystic spaces are filled with a blue-staining material. Predigestion of the section with hyaluronidase shows the spaces are empty, demonstrating that they had contained hyaluronic acid. (**A**, from *Ocular Pathology*, 2nd edn, by M Yanoff and BS Fine; **B**, AMP.)

Bibliography

Alvarado J, Murphy C, Juster R: Trabecular meshwork cellularity in primary open-angle glaucoma and nonglaucomatous normals. Ophthalmology 91:564, 1984.

Chandler PA: Narrow-angle glaucoma. Arch Ophthalmol 47:695, 1952.

Eagle RC Jr, et al: Proliferative endotheliopathy with iris abnormalities. The iridocorneal endothelial syndrome. Arch Ophthalmol 97:2014, 1979.

Fine BS, Yanoff M, Stone RA: A clinicopathologic study of four cases of primary open-angle glaucoma compared to normal eyes. Am J Ophthalmol 91:88, 1981.

Hoskins HD Jr, Shaffer RN, Hetherington J: Anatomical classification of the developmental glaucomas. Arch Ophthalmol 102:1331, 1984.

Jakobiec FA, et al: Solitary iris nevus with peripheral anterior synechias and iris endothelialization: a variant of the iris nevus syndrome. Am J Ophthalmol 83:884, 1977.

Quigley HA, et al: Blood vessels of the glaucomatous optic disc in experimental primate and human eyes. Invest Ophthalmol Vis Sci 25:918, 1984.

Rodrigues MM, Streeten BW, Spaeth GL: Chandler's syndrome as a variant of essential iris atrophy. A clinicopathologic study. Arch Ophthalmol 96:643, 1978.

Scheie HG, Yanoff M, Kellogg WT: Essential iris atrophy: report of a case. Arch Ophthalmol 94:1315, 1976.

Sugar S: Pigmentary glaucoma and the glaucoma associated with the exfoliation-pseudoexfoliation syndrome: update. Ophthalmology 91:307, 1984.

Yanoff M, Scheie HG: Melanomalytic glaucoma: report of patient. Arch Ophthalmol 84:471, 1970.

OCULAR MELANOTIC TUMORS 17

Ocular melanocytes, derived from the neural crest, are present in the eyelids, the conjunctiva, the uvea, and the pigment epithelium. Dermal melanocytes, conjunctival melanocytes, and uveal melanocytes tend to be solitary and dendritic. Pigment epithelial cells, however, form sheets of cuboidal cells which contain large, easily visualized pigment granules; this is unlike the fine, barely visualized dust-like, melanin granules of the uveal melanocytes. While pigment epithelial cells readily undergo reactive proliferation, they rarely become neoplastic. Conversely, dermal, conjunctival, and uveal melanocytes almost never undergo reactive proliferation but do give rise to neoplastic processes.

Medulloepitheliomas (previously called diktyomas) most commonly arise from the ciliary epithelium; they may also arise from pigment epithelium elsewhere, and even from the optic nerve. Medulloepitheliomas are tumors composed of elements that closely resemble the primitive medulloepithelium. They may be benign or malignant. The benign and the malignant forms may each contain heteroplastic elements (e.g., cartilage or brain-like tissue); in this case, they are called teratoid medulloepitheliomas.

In general, congenital pigmented ocular lesions fall into three categories: 1) ocular melanocytosis; 2) oculodermal melanocytosis (nevus of Ota); and 3) nevi. All three have a nevus component and may give rise in adult life to melanomas. In ocular melanocytosis, the melanoma arises in the uveal tract. In oculodermal melanocytosis, the melanoma arises in the uveal tract or skin. (Although oculodermal melanocytosis is most common in blacks and in orientals, it is rare for it to progress to a melanoma except in whites.) In nevi, the melanoma may arise in the skin, the conjunctiva, or the uvea. A rare, congenital nevus involving the optic nerve head is called a melanocytoma or magnocellular nevus. Very rarely, this can give rise to a melanoma. Melanocytomas also may arise in the uveal tract.

Acquired pigmented tumors are unusual in ocular structures. Acquired melanosis arises in the conjunctiva generally during the fifth and sixth decades of life. It may give rise to a melanoma. Adenomas and adenocarcinomas, both incidentially pigmented, may arise from the pigment epithelium of the ciliary body or iris. Fuchs' adenoma arises from the nonpigmented ciliary epithelium of the pars plicata and is a reactive lesion rather than a neoplastic one (see Chapter 9). Melanoma of the uveal tract is the most common malignant primary intraocular tumor. Melanomas may arise from preexisting nevi, as mentioned above, or may arise de novo.

Fig. 17.1 CONGENITAL MELANOCYTIC LESIONS

Ocular melanocytosis

Oculodermal melanocytosis
(nevus of Ota)

Nevi

Skin

Conjunctiva

Uvea

Medulloepithelioma

Melanocytoma (magnocellular nevus)

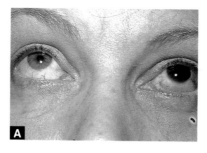

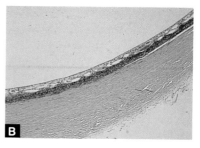

Fig. 17.2   Congenital Oculodermal Melanocytosis (Nevus of Ota).
A The patient has heterochromia (the left iris is darker than the right) and increased pigmentation of the left eyelids and sclera. **B** The patient from whom the eye illustrated here was removed (because of secondary closed-angle glaucoma) had congenital ocular melanocytosis; this eye was the involved eye. The histologic section shows hyperpigmentation of the choroid, secondary to a diffuse, maximally pigmented, choroidal nevus characteristic of the uveal lesion in congenital ocular melanocytosis.

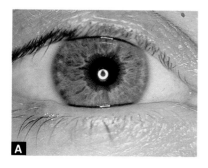

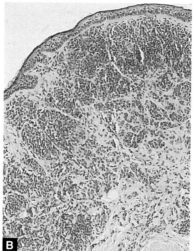

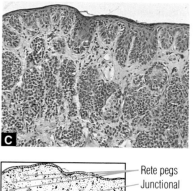

Rete pegs
Junctional nevus activity
Intradermal nests of nevus cells

Fig. 17.3   Nevus. A A lightly pigmented lesion is present at the outer aspect of the lid margin of the right lower lid. **B** A histologic section shows that the nests of nevus cells are confined to the dermis, and so is called an intradermal nevus. The nevus cells have a tendency to become smaller the deeper they appear in the dermis (this is the normal polarity). **C** In another case, nests of nevus cells are present both within the dermis and in the junctional region between epidermis and dermis, thus forming a compound nevus. Rarely, nevus cells may be present only at the junctional region, producing a junctional nevus. Malignant melanomas appear to arise only from the junctional component. (**C**, from *Ocular Pathology*, 2nd edn, by M Yanoff and BS Fine.)

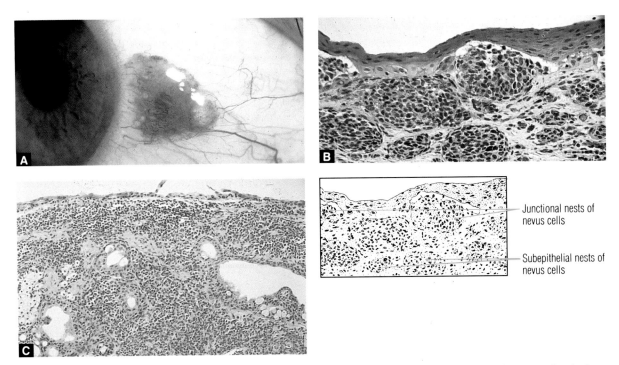

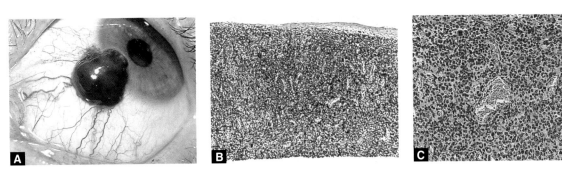

Fig. 17.4 Conjunctival Nevus. A The conjunctival nevus near the limbus shows variable pigmentation and small and large cystic structures. **B** A histologic section of another case shows nevus cells in the junctional region between the epithelial and subepithelial tissues (the substantia propria), producing a junctional nevus. As in the skin, the nevus cells tend to become smaller the deeper they are in the subepithelial tissue, representing the normal polarity of the nevus. **C** In addition to nevus cells, epithelial-lined cysts are present. These cysts often are found within the nevus and are part of the hamartomatous lesion. The cysts may be noted clinically, as seen in **A**. (**A**, from *Ocular Pathology*, 2nd edn, by M Yanoff and BS Fine.)

Fig. 17.5 Malignant Melanoma. A A pigmented conjunctival lesion near the limbus, present since childhood, had undergone recent, rapid growth. **B** A histological section of an incomplete excisional biopsy shows a heavily pigmented tumor. **C** A bleached section shows a loss of the normal polarity, i.e., the cells deep in the lesion are of the same size as those nearer the surface (instead of being smaller). Generally, melanomas not thicker than 1.5 mm have an excellent prognosis, whereas those thicker than that tend to be lethal.

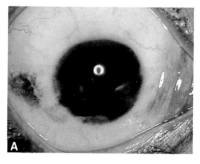

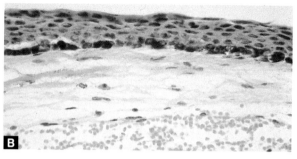

Fig. 17.6   Benign Acquired Melanosis. A The patient noted the onset of pigmentation of the conjunctiva in adult life. **B** A histological section of a biopsy of the lesion shows increased epithelial pigmentation, most marked in the basal layer, but also scattered throughout the epithelial layers. Benign acquired melanosis may resemble this or may show benign, pigmented nevus cells in the junctional position (see Fig. 17.7C).

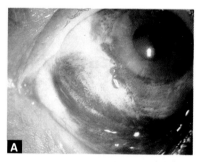

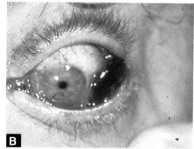

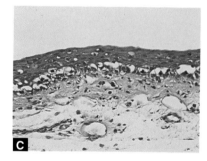

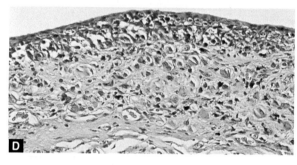

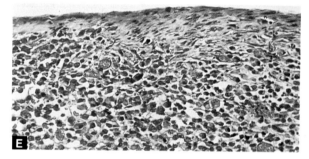

Fig. 17.7   Cancerous Acquired Melanosis. A The patient developed unilateral onset of conjunctival pigmentation in adult life. The pigmentation was completely flat. As long as the pigmentation is flat, it is unlikely that a melanoma is present. **B** This patient also had adult-onset increased conjunctival pigmentation. Recently, a mass has developed, and an excisional biopsy was performed. **C** Some areas of the lesion showed benign acquired melanosis, as represented here by nests of nevus cells in the junctional position. **D** Other areas showed cancerous melanosis, here at an early stage showing invasion of the superficial subepithelial tissue. **E** Still other areas showed frank malignant melanoma characterized by deep invasion of the subepithelial tissue. The cells are large and atypical; they show no tendency for maturation, or for following the normal cell-size polarity demonstrated in earlier figures. (**B**, from *Ocular Pathology*, 2nd edn, by M Yanoff and BS Fine.)

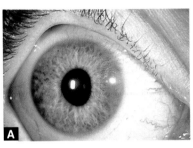

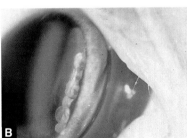

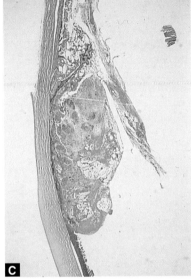

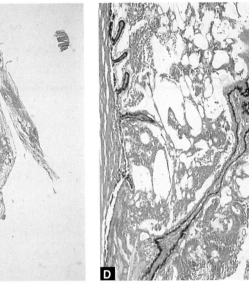

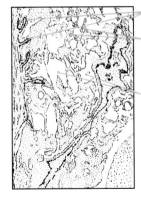

Fig. 17.9   Benign Medulloepithelioma. A The tumor seen in the anterior chamber angle nasally had originated in the ciliary body, best seen in **B** (after pupillary dilatation). **C** A histologic section of another case shows structures which resemble primitive medullary epithelium, ciliary epithelium, and retina. The tumor arises from nonpigmented ciliary epithelium. **D** Increased magnification shows the tubules of cells. Structures analogous to external limiting membrane of the retina appear on one surface of the tubules (in some areas forming lumina), while the less well defined opposite surface is in contact with a primitive vitreous. (**A, B**, courtesy of Dr. JA Shields; **C, D**, courtesy of Dr. JS McGavic.)

Ciliary process
Tubules of cells containing lumina
Primitive vitreous

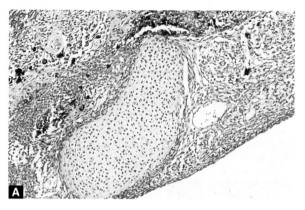

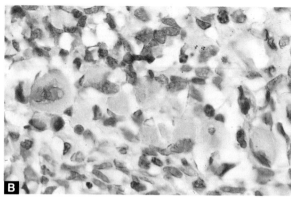

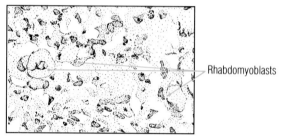

Fig. 17.10 Malignant Teratoid Medulloepithelioma.
A A heteroplastic element, namely a large nodule of
cartilage, is present within the tumor. Many atypical
cells which simulate retinoblastoma surround the
cartilage. **B** In another area, rhabdomyoblasts are
present. (Case presented by Dr. BW Streeten at the
Eastern Ophthalmic Pathology Society, 1973 and
reported by Carrillo R, Streeten BW: Arch
Ophthalmol 97:695, 1979; **A** from *Ocular Pathology*,
2nd edn, by M Yanoff and BS Fine.)

Rhabdomyoblasts

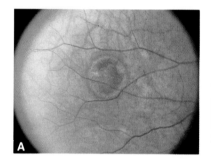

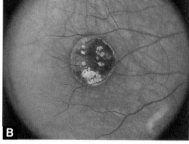

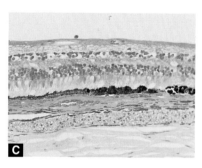

Fig. 17.11 Retinal Pigment Epithelial Hypertrophy. A The
characteristic jet-black lesion, surrounded by a halo, contains yellow
patches of irregular size and shape. **B** The same lesion, 6 years later, has
increased in size and changed in appearance. **C** A histologic section of
another case shows a sudden transition from normal retinal pigment
epithelium (RPE) to one with markedly enlarged cells. The enlarged cells
contain enlarged pigment granules (called macromelanosomes). Often, at
the edge of such a lesion, the RPE cells are depigmented, giving rise to
the halo seen clinically around the lesion. (**C** presented by Dr. WR Lee at
the European Ophthalmic Pathology Society meeting in Germany, 1982.)

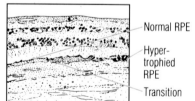

Normal RPE

Hyper-
trophied
RPE

Transition

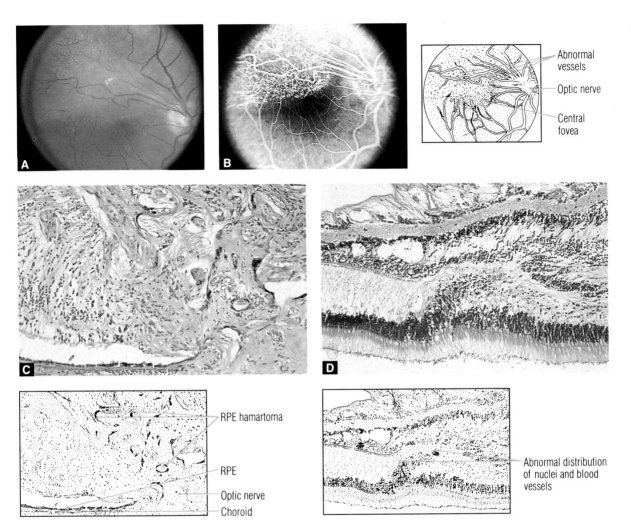

Fig. 17.12 Hamartoma of the Retinal Pigment Epithelium. A A 23-year-old nurse had esotropia of the right eye since childhood. Examination shows a thickened retina superior to the fovea. A few specks of what appears to be calcium are present in the lesion. **B** Fluorescein angiography shows a highly vascularized lesion which contains abnormal blood vessels. **C** A histologic section of another case shows that the RPE has proliferated into the retina in the juxtapapillary area. Both proliferating pigmented cells and abnormal retinal blood vessels are seen. **D** In another area, an abnormal extension of the outer nuclear layer reaches into the outer plexiform layer, along with abnormally located small blood vessels. (Case in **C** and **D** courtesy of Dr. E Howes, and reported by Vogel MH, et al: Doc Ophthalmol 26:461, 1969.)

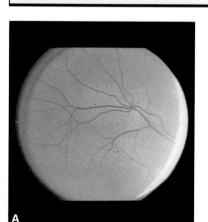

Fig. 17.15 Nevus and Adenoma. A A round, pigmented nevus is present in the fundus. The nevus contains scattered drusen on its surface superiorly. Nevi are quite common, found in the ciliary body and choroid in one eye in about 30% of patients. **B** A histologic section from another case shows two benign lesions, an adenoma which arises from the ciliary epithelium and a nevus of the choroid. **C** Increased magnification of the nevus shows plump, polyhedral nevus cells along with slender spindle nevus cells. The sparing of the choriocapillaris is characteristic. **D** The adenoma has a papillary appearance. The tumor is composed of chords of predominantly nonpigmented epithelial cells, but some pigmented cells also are present. **E** Alcian blue stain, for acid mucopolysaccharides, shows a positive reaction. The blue color was not observed when the unstained sections were treated with hyaluronidase prior to alcian blue staining, signifying that the material is hyaluronic acid.

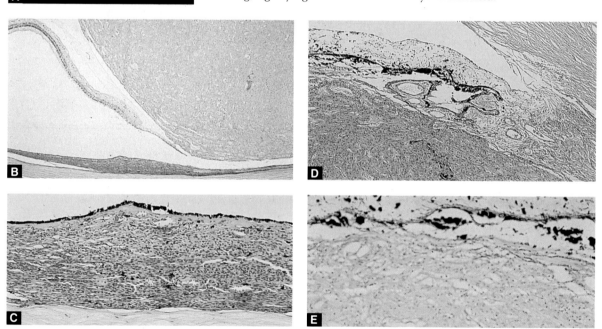

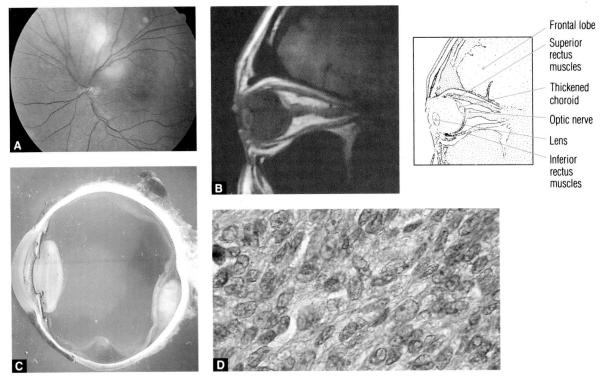

Frontal lobe
Superior rectus muscles
Thickened choroid
Optic nerve
Lens
Inferior rectus muscles

Fig. 17.16   Choroidal Malignant Melanoma. A The patient had a slowly enlarging choroidal tumor which was followed for over a 9 year period. **B** Magnetic resonance imaging (mainly T$_1$) shows the choroidal tumor just above the optic nerve. Mainly T$_2$ imaging showed that the tumor became less white, which is characteristic of a malignant melanoma (a hemangioma of the choroid, for example, becomes more white with T$_2$ imaging). **C** The enucleated eye shows the gross appearance of the tumor. **D** A histologic section demonstrates a malignant melanoma of the spindle B type.

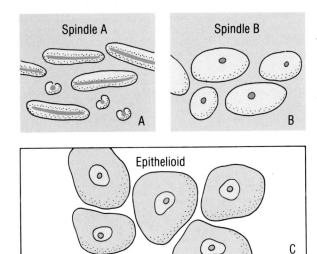

Fig. 17.17   Uveal Melanoma Cell Types. A Spindle A cells are shown in longitudinal and transverse cross sections. The cells are cohesive and have ill-defined cell borders. The nuclei contain nuclear folds that appear as dark stripes parallel to the long axis of the nuclei. The stripe is caused by an infolding of the nucleus, as noted in cross section. **B** Spindle B nuclei are larger and plumper than spindle A nuclei and contain prominent nucleoli rather than nuclear folds. The cells, similar to spindle A, are cohesive and have ill-defined cell borders. **C** Epithelioid cells are not cohesive, have distinct cell borders, and show large, oval nuclei which contain prominent nucleoli. The cells are larger than spindle A and spindle B cells.

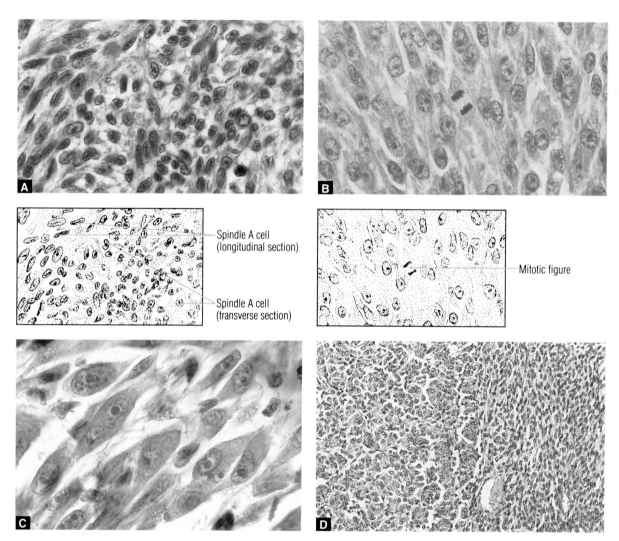

Spindle A cell
(longitudinal section)

Spindle A cell
(transverse section)

Mitotic figure

Fig. 17.18   Uveal Melanoma Cells. A Spindle A cells, identified by their dark stripe parallel to the long axis of the nucleus, are seen in longitudinal section. They are identified in transverse cross section by the infolding of the nuclear membrane that causes the dark stripe. **B** Spindle B cells are identified by their prominent nucleoli. Note the mitotic figure. Both spindle A and spindle B cells tend to be quite cohesive and have ill-defined cell borders. **C** Epithelioid cells are the largest of the melanoma cells, tend not to be cohesive, and have irregular shapes and sizes and very prominent nucleoli within the large nuclei. **D** Some melanomas contain a mixture of spindle cells and epithelioid cells. The left half of this figure is occupied by epithelioid cells and the right half by spindle cells (this is called a mixed-cell type melanoma).

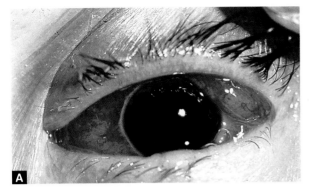

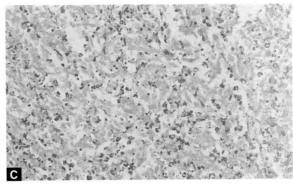

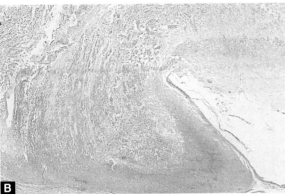

Fig. 17.19 Necrotic Uveal Melanoma. A The patient presented with recent onset of blindness, pain, redness, and chemosis. Examination by ultrasonography showed a solid tumor. The eye was enucleated. B A histologic section shows that the typical "mushroom" tumor had undergone spontaneous necrosis, making identification of the melanoma cell type almost impossible. This type, shown with increased magnification in C, is therefore called the necrotic cell type melanoma. Completely necrotic melanomas often present clinically as this patient did, with the appearance of inflammation.

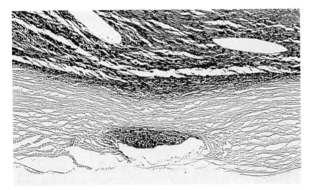

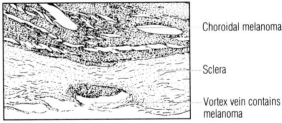

Choroidal melanoma

Sclera

Vortex vein contains melanoma

Fig. 17.20 Vortex Vein Invasion. A large, pigmented, choroidal melanoma is present within the eye and is filling most of an intrascleral vortex vein.

(From *Ocular Pathology,* 2nd edn, by M Yanoff and BS Fine.)

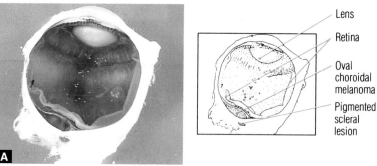

Fig. 17.21 Extraocular Extension. A Note the oval, pigmented melanoma of the choroid within the eye and the small pigmented lesion on the surface of the sclera. **B** A histologic section shows the uveal melanoma within the eye and a nodule of extrascleral extension.

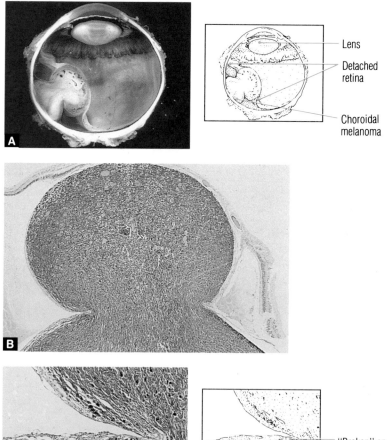

Fig. 17.22 Uveal "Mushroom" Melanoma. A The melanoma has ruptured through Bruch's membrane, causing a mushroom configuration. The elastic Bruch's membrane remains around the base of the mushroom, acting as a tourniquet. Arteriolar blood gains access to the head of the mushroom, but venous blood has difficulty leaving, giving rise to dilated, engorged blood vessels in the head of the mushroom, as noted here. **B** A histologic section shows the ruptured ends of Bruch's membrane (seen with increased magnification in **C**) and the dilated, engorged blood vessels in the head of the tumor.

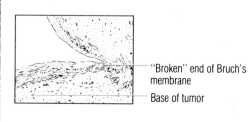

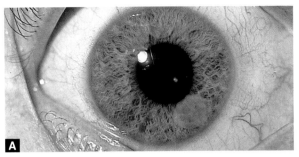

Fig. 17.23 Iris Melanoma. A A lightly pigmented, vascularized tumor is present in the iris inferonasally. The tumor has caused some blunting of the pupillary border in that region. **B** A histologic section shows spindle melanoma cells "spilling" over the pupillary border. **C** The cells invade the stroma of the iris. Often, as in this case, the spindle cells appear different from ciliary body and choroidal spindle A and B cells, and seem to be more benign.

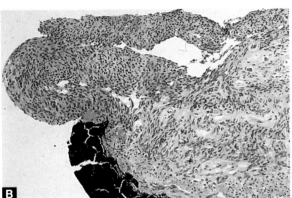

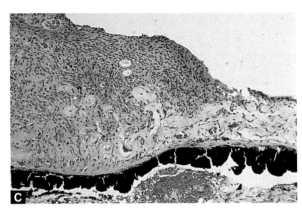

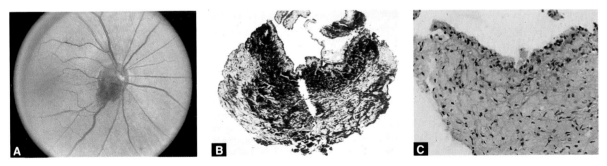

FIG. 17.24 MELANOCYTOMA (magnocellular nevus)

Optic nerve head   Uvea

Fig. 17.25 Melanocytoma. A Melanocytoma of the optic disc characteristically is black in color, has an inferior temporal location, and contains feathered edges. Similar tumors may occur in the choroid and ciliary body. **B** A histologic section of a ciliary body melanocytoma shows that the tumor is composed of maximally pigmented nevus cells. **C** A bleached section shows benign, plump, polyhedral nevus cells. A melanocytoma is simply a nevus that is composed entirely of maximally pigmented, polyhedral nevus cells. (Case in **B** and **C** reported by Scheie HG and Yanoff M: Arch Ophthalmol 77:81, 1967.)

Bibliography

Brownstein S, et al: Nonteratoid medulloepithelioma of the ciliary body. Ophthalmology 91:1118, 1984.

Cantrill HL, et al: Retinal vascular changes in malignant melanoma of the choroid. Am J Ophthalmol 97:411, 1984.

Carrillo R, Streeten BW: Malignant teratoid medulloepithelioma in an adult. Arch Ophthalmol 97:695, 1979.

Chang M, Zimmerman LE, McLean I: The persisting pseudomelanoma problem. Arch Ophthalmol 102:726, 1984.

Folberg R, et al: Comparison of direct and microslide pathology measurements of uveal melanomas. Invest Ophthalmol Vis Sci 86:1788, 1985.

Folberg R, McLean IW, Zimmerman LE: Conjunctival melanosis and melanoma. Ophthalmology 91:673, 1984.

Frangieh GT, et al: Melanocytoma of the ciliary body: presentation of four cases and review of nineteen reports. Surv Ophthalmol 29:328, 1985.

Gass JDM: Comparison of uveal melanoma growth rates with mitotic index and mortality. Arch Ophthalmol 103:924, 1985.

Geisse LJ, Robertson DM: Iris melanomas. Am J Ophthalmol 99:638, 1985.

Holbach L, Völker HE, Naumann GOH: Malignes teratoides Medulloepitheliom des Ziliarkörpers und saures Gliafaserprotein. Klinische, histochemische und immunohistochemische Befunde. Klin Mbl Augenheilk 187:282, 1985.

Kersten RC, Tse DT, Anderson R: Iris melanoma. Nevus or malignancy? Surv Ophthalmol 29:423, 1985.

Naumann G, Zimmerman LE, Yanoff M: Histogenesis of malignant melanomas of the uvea. I. Histopathologic characteristics of nevi of the choroid and ciliary body. Arch Ophthalmol 76:784, 1966.

Papale JJ, et al: Adenocarcinoma of the ciliary body pigment epithelium in a child. Arch Ophthalmol 102:100, 1984.

Rajpal S, Moore R, Karakousis CP: Survival in metastatic ocular melanoma. Cancer 52:334, 1983.

Reidy JJ, et al: Melanocytoma: nomenclature, pathogenesis, natural history and treatment (Review). Surv Ophthalmol 29:319, 1985.

Schachat AP, et al: Combined hamartomas of the retina and retinal pigment epithelium. Ophthalmology 91:1609, 1984.

Scheie HG, Yanoff M: Pseudomelanoma of ciliary body, report of a patient. Arch Ophthalmol 77:81, 1967.

Shields CL, et al: Differentiation of adenoma of the iris pigment epithelium from iris cyst and melanoma. Am J Ophthalmol 100:678, 1985.

Velazquez N, Jones IS: Ocular and oculodermal melanocytosis associated with uveal melanoma. Ophthalmology 90:1472, 1983.

Vogel MH, Zimmerman LE, Gass JDM: Proliferation of the juxtapapillary retinal pigment epithelium simulating malignant melanoma. Doc Ophthalmol 26:461, 1969.

Wang C-L, Brucker AJ: Vitreous hemorrhage secondary to juxtapapillary vascular hamartoma of the retina. Retina 4:44, 1984.

Yanoff M, Zimmerman LE: Histogenesis of malignant melanoma of the uvea. II. Relationship of uveal nevi to malignant melanomas. Cancer 20:493, 1967.

Zimmerman LE, McLean IW: Do growth and onset of symptoms of uveal melanomas indicate subclinical metastasis? Ophthalmology 91:685, 1984.

RETINOBLASTOMA 18

Retinoblastoma is one of the most common childhood malignancies. It is the most common malignant intraocular childhood neoplasm and follows only uveal melanomas and metastatic carcinomas as the most common human intraocular malignancy. The frequency is approximately 1 in 18,000 live births. The average age at the time of initial diagnosis is 13 months; 89% are diagnosed before 3 years of age.

Retinoblastoma in affected families behaves as an autosomal dominant mendelian trait that has incomplete penetrance and variable expressivity. The normal allele at chromosome band 13q14 acts as a mendelian dominant. If one of the two alleles normally found at this site is absent, as may occur in the chromosome 13 deletion syndrome, retinoblastoma will still not develop unless a second "hit" occurs that makes the individual homozygous with respect to the absence of the normal allele. Familial (inherited) cases constitute 10% of the total incidence of retinoblastoma; 90% of the cases are sporadic. Among the sporadic cases, 25% arise as mutations in the germ line and, therefore, will become hereditable. The rest of the cases arise as a result of mutations in the somatic (retinal) cells and cannot be inherited. Bilateral retinoblastoma, as well as multifocal retinoblastoma in one eye, generally are caused by inherited retinoblastoma. Retinoblastoma may arise simultaneously and primarily in both eyes and in the pineal gland; this is called trilateral retinoblastoma.

At the cellular level, retinoblastomas are quite primitive and undifferentiated. Structures, such as Flexner–Wintersteiner and Homer Wright rosettes, as well as fleurettes, may be found. A patient whose tumor has abundant Flexner–Wintersteiner rosettes has about a six-fold better prognosis than a patient whose tumor has no rosettes. A tumor composed entirely of fleurettes also indicates an excellent prognosis. The mortality rate is around 25% if the tumor invades the choroid slightly; this rises to 65% when the invasion is massive. When the tumor does not invade the optic nerve, the mortality rate is approximately 8%. If invasion extends to the lamina cribosa, but not beyond, the mortality rate rises to around 15%. When the invasion is posterior to the lamina cribosa, but not in the cut end of the nerve, the mortality rate is about 44%. If the invasion is to the point of surgical transection or to the posterior point of exit of the central retinal vessels from the optic nerve, the mortality rate is about 65%. Unfortunately, even when the retinoblastoma is "cured", a significant proportion of patients will develop a second malignancy, which may prove fatal. The increased incidence of second malignancies, especially osteosarcoma, is not necessarily related to radiation therapy undergone in the treatment of the primary retinoblastoma.

Retinoblastomas often present clinically with a cat's eye reflex, called leukokoria. A number of conditions may mimic retinoblastoma and also present with leukokoria; these are called pseudogliomas (the old term for retinoblastoma was glioma, hence the term pseudoglioma). The most common pseudogliomas are persistent hyperplastic primary vitreous, retinal dysplasia (most often associated with 13 trisomy—see Chapter 2), retinopathy of prematurity, toxocara endophthalmitis, and Coats' disease. Not only may the pseudogliomas present with leukokoria, they also may present as localized, small lesions resembling those of retinoblastoma.

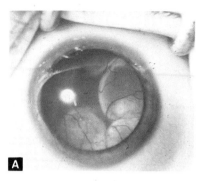 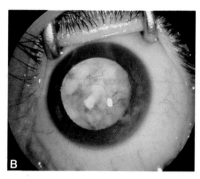 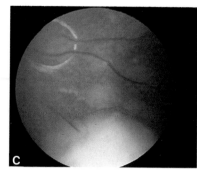

Fig. 18.1   Retinoblastoma. A Retinoblastomas may arise mainly from the external retinal layers, grow externally (exophytic growth), and cause a retinal detachment. This patient, who presented with leukokoria, had a solid tumor under the retinal detachment. **B** Retinoblastomas may grow predominantly from the inner layers of the retina (endophytic growth) into the vitreous. Their clinical appearance, as here, closely resembles that of brain tissue. Often, the retinoblastoma arises at different levels of the retina and grows both inward and outward. **C** The retinoblastoma may grow as individual discrete retinal tumors. Here we see two small tumors and one large tumor inferiorly. (**A, B,** courtesy of Dr. HG Scheie, and from *Ocular Pathology*, 2nd edn, by M Yanoff and BS Fine; **C,** courtesy of Dr. DB Schaffer.)

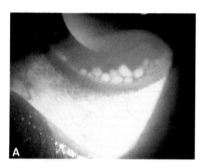

Fig. 18.2   Retinoblastoma. A Retinoblastoma cells have formed balls of tumor in the anterior chamber inferiorly, simulating a hypopyon, thus "pseudohypopyon". **B** Iris neovascularization may arise secondary to the retinal process. The iris neovascularization can lead to peripheral anterior synechiae and a secondary closed-angle glaucoma. In infants, this may give rise to buphthalmos (as occurred here). **C** Rarely, the retinoblastoma, if untreated, may invade the orbit and result in proptosis. (**A,** courtesy of Dr. AJ Shields; **B,** courtesy of Dr. HG Scheie, and from *Ocular Pathology*, 2nd edn, by M Yanoff and BS Fine; **C,** courtesy of Dr. RE Shannon.)

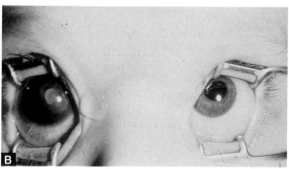 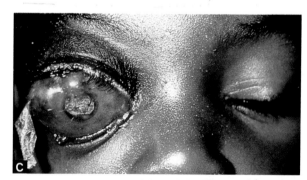

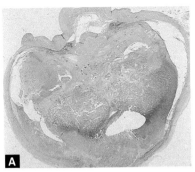

Fig. 18.3 Retinoblastoma. A Characteristically, sections of retinoblastoma stained with hematoxylin and eosin and viewed under low magnification, show some dark blue areas, surrounded by light pink areas. The dark areas represent the viable cells and calcium deposition, and the light areas represent tumor necrosis. **B** Increased magnification shows viable (dark blue) tumor cells clustered around central blood vessels, and themselves surrounded by a mantle of necrotic (pink) cells. Numerous Flexner–Wintersteiner rosettes are present. **C** Further increased magnification shows the viable tumor cells around blood vessels, the necrotic areas, and the Flexner–Wintersteiner rosettes.

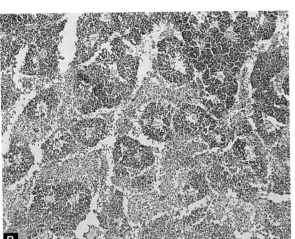

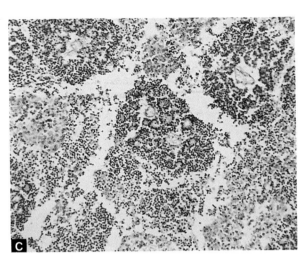

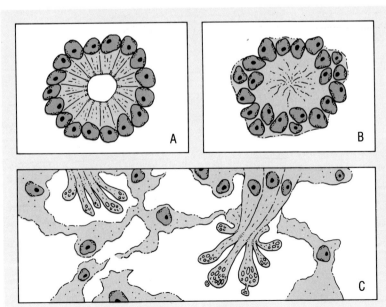

Fig. 18.4 Types of Rosettes. A The Flexner–Wintersteiner rosette consists of a central lumen lined by cuboidal tumor cells that contain nuclei positioned basally (away from the lumen). Delicate limiting membranes are seen at the apices of the cells which surround the lumen. **B** Homer Wright rosettes are found more frequently in medulloblastomas and neuroblastomas than in retinoblastomas. In these rosettes, the cells line up around an acellular area which contains cobweb-like material. **C** Fleurettes are flower-like groupings of tumor cells within the retinoblastoma. The cells of fleurettes show clear evidence of differentiation into photoreceptor elements.

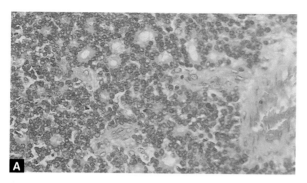

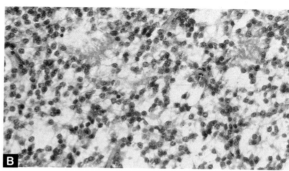

Fig. 18.5 Rosettes and Fleuretttes. A Flexner–Wintersteiner rosettes show clear lumina lined by a delicate limiting membrane and cuboidal retinoblastoma cells with basally oriented nuclei. **B** In this histologic section of a retinoblastoma, almost all of the cells show photoreceptor differentiation, indicated by the pale, eosinophilic acellular regions. The differentiated areas are forming fleurettes.

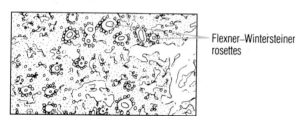

Flexner–Wintersteiner rosettes

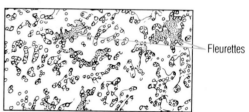

Fleurettes

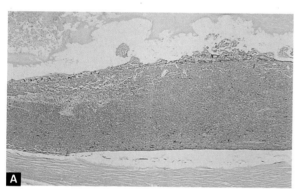

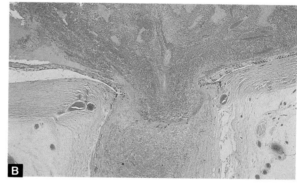

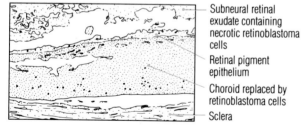

Subneural retinal exudate containing necrotic retinoblastoma cells

Retinal pigment epithelium

Choroid replaced by retinoblastoma cells

Sclera

Fig. 18.6 Invasion by Retinoblastoma. A The retinoblastoma has invaded through Bruch's membrane, massively replacing the choroid. Among patients with mild invasion of the choroid, there is a 25% mortality rate. Those with massive invasion, as shown here, have a mortality rate of about 65%. **B** The retinoblastoma has invaded the optic nerve up to the cut end. For those patients in whom the substance of the optic nerve has been invaded posterior to the lamina cribosa, the mortality rate is around 44%. If retinoblastoma is present at the cut end of the optic nerve, the mortality rate is approximately 65%.

FIG. 18.7 PSEUDOGLIOMAS—LEUKOKORIA

Persistent hyperplastic primary vitreous (PHPV)
Retinal dysplasia (see Chapter 2)
Retinopathy of prematurity
Toxocara endophthalmitis
Coats' disease
Norrie's disease
Incontinentia pigmenti
Massive retinal fibrosis
Metastatic retinitis
Congenital nonattachment of the retina
Secondary retinal detachment
Juvenile retinoschisis (see Chapter 11)
Embryonal medulloepithelioma (see Chapter 17)

FIG. 18.8 PERSISTENT HYPERPLASTIC PRIMARY VITREOUS

Congenital and unilateral   Long ciliary processes
Present at birth   Persistent hyaloid artery
Microphthalmos   Lens capsule dehiscence
Shallow anterior chamber

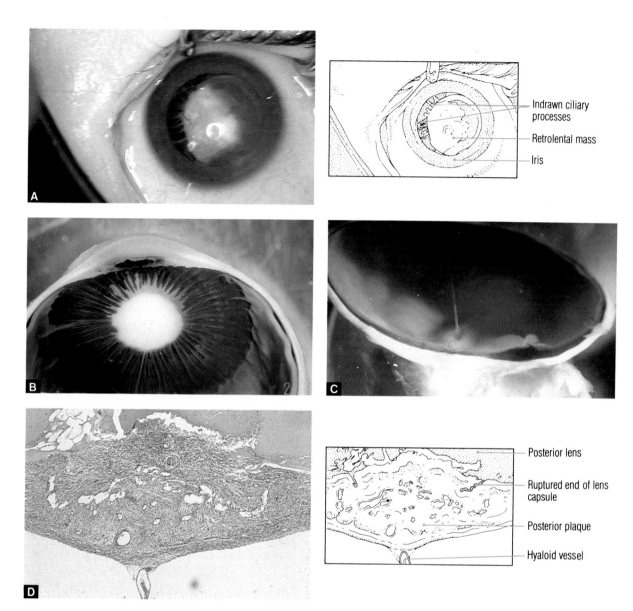

With labels: Indrawn ciliary processes, Retrolental mass, Iris; Posterior lens, Ruptured end of lens capsule, Posterior plaque, Hyaloid vessel

Fig. 18.9   Persistent Hyperplastic Primary Vitreous (PHPV). A Clinically, characteristically the ciliary processes are drawn inward and a posterior lens opacity is noted. **B, C** Gross specimens of another case show a persistent hyaloid vessel and the ciliary processes stretched inward toward a posterior lens plaque (**B**); in **C** the hyaloid vessel extends to the optic nerve. **D** A histologic section shows abundant mesenchymal fibrovascular tissue just behind and within the posterior lens. Note the ends of the ruptured lens capsule. A persistent hyaloid vessel also is present. (**A** from *Ocular Pathology*, 2nd edn, by M Yanoff and BS Fine; **B, C, D**, courtesy of Dr. BW Streeten and reported in Caudill JW, Streeten BW, Tso MOM: Opthalmology 92:1153, 1985.)

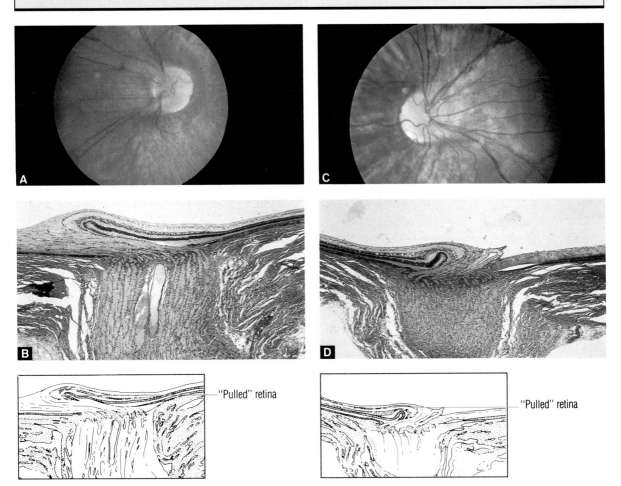

FIG. 18.10 RETINOPATHY OF PREMATURITY

Not congenital*   **Related to prematurity and oxygen administration**

Not present at birth

Eyes normal size at birth but
  may become microphthalmic

*Atypical forms may be present at birth.

"Pulled" retina

"Pulled" retina

Fig. 18.11 Retinopathy of Prematurity (ROP).
A The fundus picture shows the blood vessels in this right eye pulled temporally. **B** A histologic section of another right eye shows the nasal retina displaced temporally over the optic nerve head. **C** This is the clinical appearance of the left eye of the patient shown in **A**. **D** A histologic section of another left eye (from the patient shown in **B**), demonstrates the temporal pulling of the nasal retina. (**A–D**, from *Ocular Pathology*, 2nd edn, by M Yanoff and BS Fine.)

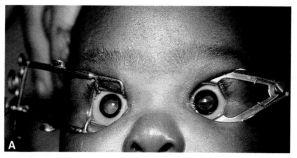

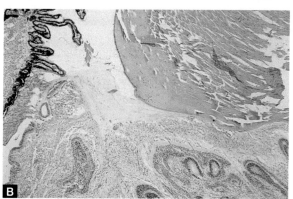

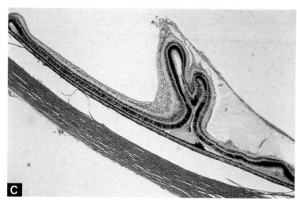

Fig. 18.12   ROP. A A 6-month-old baby shows bilateral leukokoria secondary to ROP. **B** A histologic section of another eye shows the detached retina drawn by fibrovascular tissue into a mass behind the lens (hence, the old term of retrolental fibroplasia). **C** Neovascularization of the retina has occurred anterior to the equator, forming fibrovascular bands, and causing a traction detachment of the retina. (**A**, from *Ocular Pathology*, 2nd edn, by M Yanoff and BS Fine.)

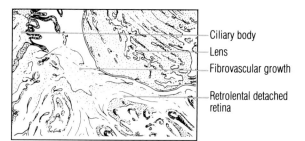

Ciliary body
Lens
Fibrovascular growth
Retrolental detached retina

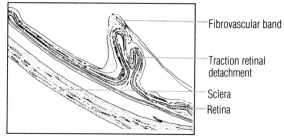

Fibrovascular band
Traction retinal detachment
Sclera
Retina

FIG. 18.13 TOXOCARIASIS (*Toxocara canis*)

Ocular manifestation of visceral larva migrans
Involves children 6 to 11 years of age
Two forms: leukokoria and discrete lesions
Zonal granulomatous reaction around eosinophilic abscess and
    worm

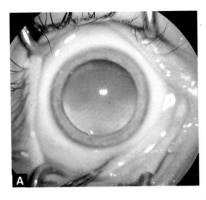

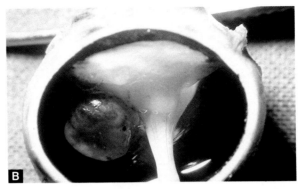

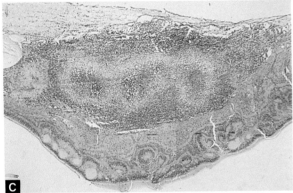

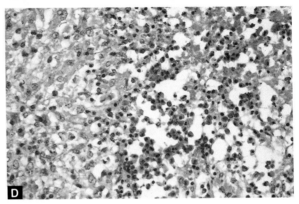

Fig. 18.14 Toxocariasis. A This 8-year-old boy presented with leukokoria. The eye was white; other than loss of vision, no additional symptoms were present. **B** Another eye displaying leukokoria was enucleated to rule out retinoblastoma. **C** A histologic section shows a peripheral retinal mass which contains an eosinophilic abscess. **D** Increased magnification shows a collection of eosinophils which are surrounded by a chronic, granulomatous, inflammatory reaction. Often, the worm itself is not found, but the eosinophils are evidence for its presence prior to dissolution.

Fig. 18.15 COATS' DISEASE

Unilateral
Occurs mainly between the ages of 8 months to 18 years
Two-thirds occur in male children
Retinal telangiectasis is the earliest sign
Exudative, bullous retinal detachment may be end result

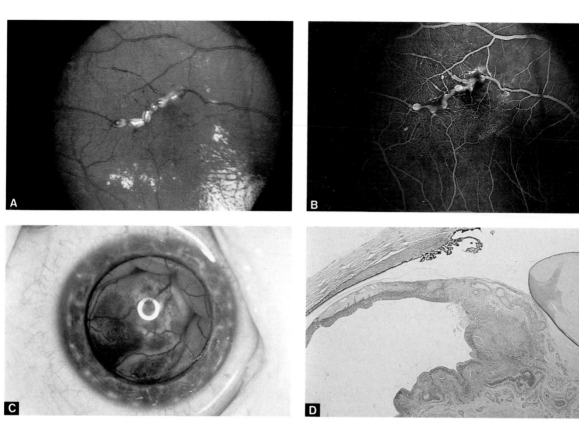

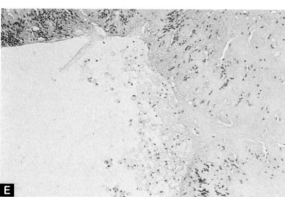

Fig. 18.16 Coats' Disease. A Abnormal, telangiectatic retinal vessels show the typical "light bulb" appearance. These vessels leak fluid into and under the neural retina. **B** Fluorescein angiography of the same case shows the abnormal telangiectatic vessels. **C** The exudation may increase and result in an exudative retinal detachment, as occurred in this case. Note the telangiectatic vessels on the surface of the retina. **D** A histologic section of another case shows large, telangiectatic vessels in the peripheral retina. The vessels have leaked fluid, especially into the outer layers of the retina, causing a spreading and necrosis of the outer retina. **E** Increased magnification shows foamy (lipoidal) histiocytes engulfing the lipid-rich exudate in the outer layers of the retina and in the subretinal space. (**C,** from *Ocular Pathology*, 2nd edn, by M Yanoff and BS Fine.)

Bibliography

Abramson DH, et al: Second nonocular tumors in retinoblastoma survivors. Are they radiation-induced? Ophthalmology 91:1351, 1984.

Brownstein S, de Chadarevian J-P, Little JM: Trilateral retinoblastoma. Report of two cases. Arch Ophthalmol 102:257, 1984.

Caudill JW, Streeten BW, Tso MOM: Phacoanaphylactoid reaction in persistent hyperplastic primary vitreous. Ophthalmology 92:1153, 1985.

Chang M, McLean IW, Merrit JC: Coats' disease—a study of 62 histologically confirmed cases. J Pediatr Ophthalmol Strabismus 21:163, 1984.

Dryja TP, et al: Homozygosity of chromosome 13 in retinoblastoma. N Engl J Med 310:550, 1984.

Font RL, Yanoff M, Zimmerman LE: Intraocular adipose tissue and persistent hyperplastic primary vitreous. Arch Ophthalmol 82:43, 1969.

Fryczkowski AW, et al: Scanning electron microscopy of the ocular vasculature in retinopathy of prematurity. Arch Ophthalmol 103:224, 1985.

Gallie BL, Phillips RA: Retinoblastoma: a model of oncogenesis. Ophthalmology 91:666, 1984.

Lee W-H, et al: Human retinoblastoma susceptibility gene: cloning, identification, and sequence. Science 235: 1394, 1987.

Lin CCL, Tso MOM: An electron microscopic study of calcification of retinoblastoma. Am J Ophthalmol 96:765, 1983.

Machemer R: Description and pathogenesis of late stages of retinopathy of prematurity. Ophthalmology 92:1000, 1985.

Patz A: Observations on the retinopathy of prematurity. Am J Ophthalmol 100:164, 1985.

Shields JA: Ocular toxocariasis. A review. Surv Ophthalmol 28:361, 1984.

Tarkkanen A, Karjalainen K: Excess of cancer deaths in close relatives of patients with bilateral retinoblastomas. Ophthalmologica 189:143, 1984.

INDEX

Page numbers in roman type refer to text; those in italics refer to tables; those in boldface refer to illustrations.